Step by Step Approach to Practice

Classical Homoeopathy

Beginner's Guide

Dr Pravin Karthikeyan

NOTION PRESS

NOTION PRESS

India. Singapore. Malaysia.

ISBN 978-1-64783-944-4

This book has been published with all reasonable efforts taken to make the material error-free after the consent of the author. No part of this book shall be used, reproduced in any manner whatsoever without written permission from the author, except in the case of brief quotations embodied in critical articles and reviews.

The Author of this book is solely responsible and liable for its content including but not limited to the views, representations, descriptions, statements, information, opinions and references ["Content"]. The Content of this book shall not constitute or be construed or deemed to reflect the opinion or expression of the Publisher or Editor. Neither the Publisher nor Editor endorse or approve the Content of this book or guarantee the reliability, accuracy or completeness of the Content published herein and do not make any representations or warranties of any kind, express or implied, including but not limited to the implied warranties of merchantability, fitness for a particular purpose. The Publisher and Editor shall not be liable whatsoever for any errors, omissions, whether such errors or omissions result from negligence, accident, or any other cause or claims for loss or damages of any kind, including without limitation, indirect or consequential loss or damage arising out of use, inability to use, or about the reliability, accuracy or sufficiency of the information contained in this book.

Dedicated to all the true learners of Homoeopathy

Contents

Foreword xi

Preface xv

Acknowledgments xvii

Introduction 1

1. Understanding the basics 9

Planes of the body 9

Dynamic Influence 13

Effect of dynamic influence on Vital force 17

Dynamic protective covering 20

Role of vital force in health 29

What makes a person sick? 31

Disease ultimates 35

Role of vital force in disease 36

Source of physical symptoms 37

Sick 40

What to expect from our remedies and where it acts? 45

2. Studying a drug from materia medica 47

In Homeopathy there are no surogates 48

Conceptual image of remedy 52

Image of sickness or portrait of disease 55

Individualization 58

Perfect Similimum 60

Basis for selection of a remedy 62

3. Suceptability, predisposition and Miasms (An introduction) 65

4. Case taking 77

Aims and objectives: In acute cases 77

Managing acute cases 78

Collecting the information in an acute case 83

Acute totality: 93

Art and skill of taking an acute case 93

Guidelines and instructions for take a case 101

Aphorism 83 101

Aphorism 84 112

Aphorism 85: 118

Aphorism 86: 119

Aphorism 87: 121

Aphorism 88: 124

Aphorism 89: 128

Aphorism 90:	129
Aphorism 91:	130
Aphorism 92:	133
Aphorism 93:	134
Aphorism 94:	138
Aphorism 95:	139
Aphorism 96:	143
Aphorism 97:	145
Aphorism 98:	148
Aphorism 99:	150
Aphorism 100:	151
Aphorism 101:	152
Aphorism 102:	153
Aphorism 103:	154
Aphorism 104:	155
5. Classification of symptoms	157
General Symptoms	164
Physical generals	170
Particular symptoms	172
Symptoms of normal disposition & changed disposition	176
Evaluation of symptoms	179
6. Case Analysis and Evaluation	183

Giving value to an observed symptom 183

Importance of studying allied subjects 188

Importance of clinical diagnosis in Homoeopathy ... 192

Totality of a case 198

Repertorial totality 198

Potential Differential Field (PDF) 199

Repertorization and Repertorial result 200

Selecting the final remedy 201

7. Boenninghausen's Thereupeutic pocket book 203

Philosophic Background 203

Plan and construction: 205

Clinical utility of BTPB 206

Method of working out a case 206

8. Boger Boenninghausen's Characteristics and Repertory (B.B.C.R) 209

Philosophical background 209

Doctrine of complete symptoms and concomitants: 210

Doctrine of pathological generals: 210

Doctrine of causation and time: 211

Clinical Rubrics: 211

Evaluation of remedies 211

Fever Totality 212

Concordances: 212

- Plan and construction 212
- Methods of Repertorization 215
- 9. Kent's Repertory 219
- Philosophic background 219
- Grading of remedies 220
- Kent's concept of totality 221
- Plan and construction 222
- Arrangement of rubrics 224
- Method of working out a case 226
  - Addition method 226
  - Eliminating method 227
- 10. General Topics 231
- Limitations of Homoeopathy 231
- Advantages of Homeopathy 232
- Obstacles to cure 234
- Difficulties in taking a chronic case 237
- Homoeopathy as medicine of future: 244
- How to approach Fever cases 247
- Do we have painkillers in Homoeopathy? 250
- Role of Homoeopathic remedies in Mechanical trauma 253
- Role of placebos in Homoeopathy 255
- Prescribing in pathological cases: 266

Polypharmacy or prescribing multiple remedies: 268

One-line prescribers: 269

Keynote prescription: 270

Listing remedies for clinical conditions: 272

Managing surgical cases: 273

Defective books and defective use of books: 274

Value of experience: 276

Consistency is the key: 278

Reference 280

Epilogue 281

Foreword

In continuation of the work done on the Mind rubrics of Kent's Repertory Dr Pravin Karthikeyan has come up with a new approach for the beginners to practice classical Homoeopathy.

Mareria medica, Philosophy and Repertory are so closely interwoven into one another that no Homoeopathic doctor can aspire to do anything worth while without the constant study of each of these disciplines and without constant reference to them.

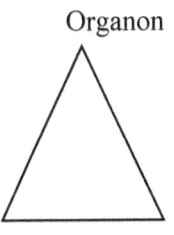

Organon

Materia Medica   Repertory

Dr Pravin Karthikeyan in this book has given this remarkable relation in easy and understandable language, which will provide abase as well as enhance the knowledge of all the three noted works by Dr Kent and Dr Hahnemann.

Dr Pravin Karthikeyan has understood the difficulties of the beginners which he must have also faced in his startup years and provided such a good book to read and understand Homoeopathy for practitioners and beginner's.

Dr Kent has written "A physician advanced in years looks back upon many failures. The faithful Homoeopathist recalls a man, a woman, a child, and realizes that these, among his past failures would now be simple cases. Prescribing the Homoeopathic remedy is such a process of growth and progress that it may be said that "The best of wine is saved for the last feast."

Dr Pravin Karthikeyan with his team has immensely put efforts to enkindle the knowledge provided by Philosophy, Organon and Materia medica and to understand them thoroughly.

May this effort be flourished, and all the Homoeopaths unite to stand and prove that Homeopathy is not just a placebo effect, but it is based on research and philosophies.

Dr Supriya Agarwal

Practitioner Lucknow

Classical homoepathy Beginner's Guide was a deep essence of homeopathy which is a 15 years experience as a teacher and practitioner of homeopathy was written by dr pravin Kartikeyan sir , since there are lots of books writing with different methodologies in today society but this book hold a unique place with all the essence taken by our basic literatures and philosophy with a continuous understanding at the level of students and practitioners professionals, Need was this book came in to light after a survey in indian collages with a huge number of students and practitioners. This book holds a full treasure of knowledge of homoeopathy.

Really this masterpiece gift by dr pravin sir will open up your mind to think over a deep essence of homeopathy science and art.

Congratulations to sir and entrie team of homeomirror which brought this book into reality to help all the beginners like students' practitioners to understand the deep essence Hahnemann's homoeopathy.

Dr Bimlesh Tiwari

Practitioner, Mumbai

Preface

The book Step by step approach to practice Classical Homoeopathy is a guide for the beginners to learn and master this wonderful art of practicing classical Homeopathy.

It is a well know fact that despite having existed for over 200 years our system still faces crtics and allegations. These critics and allegations we face are not because our system lacks the potential, but the fact is, we lack that knowledge to utilize the true potential of Homeopathy.

Today we lack unity and we are divided among us under various methodologies. Keeping in mind the growth of our system and growth of eachj one of use we have to find out a way to create a unity among us and fight together to put an end to these critics and allegations.

This unity can come only when we all have a common understanding, a common perception and a commo methodology. If we all start follwoinga common methodology, then te time shall come when we all shall unite together as a team to show to the world the true potential of Homeopathy.

So, we need to finmd out a way to sort out our own internal conflicts and differences. The conflicts and differences can be sorted out only when we learn to stick to the basic laws, theories and principles of

Homeopathy. We shoud all consider our literature as the final authority and learn to stick with the instructions and guidelines given in the literature.

Many of us tend to get deviated from this right path either because of lack of knowledge or lack of proper guidance when it was needed. This book is an attempt to give that guidance to each and every sincere learner who wishes to explore this wonderful art of healing.

It covers all necessary topics explained in a very simple and easy way that is needed for each one of us to understand before we sit out to practice. Attempt has been made to keep the language easy and simple for helping even those students who find it difficult to read and grasp from the original literature.

This book contains no new discoveries or theories, but it is strictly limited to explaining the basic concepts with the help of some interesting examples and clinical co-relations. I hope that this book shall help both the students as well as the practitioners to master this wonderful art of practicing classical homeopathy.

Dr Pravin Karthikeyan

Date: 12/11/2019

Acknowledgments

As an author the journey so far has been indeed a very challenging one. The contents included in this book has not been written overnight but has involved a lot of hard work, dedication and time. This is indeed a dream come true for me to get this opportunity to share my experience and understandings with the friends and felowmens of this great and wonderful art of healing.

I strongly believe that curiosity is the mother of all revolutions. The curuiosity first ignites your own internal conscience to hunt for the truth and understand it.Then the curiosity shifts to attaining perfection which is then followed by the curiosity to share this truth and understanding with others to ensure the same perfection is attained by each and every true healer who is proud to call themselves as a Homeopath.

I take this opportunity to sincerily thank from my heart each and every person who has laid a steppingstone for me in this journey so far. Special thanks to all the subscribed members of HOMOEOMIRROR whicout them probably this venture would have been impossible.

A very special thanks to all the LIFELONG MEMBERS of homoeomirror for their kind support extended to set up our clinic at Kochi (Kerala).

Some special personalities indeed deserve to get acknowledged specially for their esteem role in helping this project to flourish. I would tthank from my heart Dr

Chandrasekhar Pore sir who has alays been an inspiration to me.

A very special thanks to Dr Bimlesh Tiwari for holding my hands in the bad times as a brother and imparting the energy and confidence in me to wrtite this book.

At the same time i would also like to specially thank Dr Pavan Kumar, Dr Rakhi for showing such a dedication and personal interest in helping me to complete this book.

I have put in my best efforts to design this book in a very innovative and interesting way. I sincerily hope that this work shall find a place in the heart of all true lovers of Homeopathy across the world.

Introduction

It's said that Homoeopathy is a science but practicing it is an art. An art is something that cannot be taught unless one has the interest to learn and master it. Practicing Homoeopathy basically involves two steps. One is "collecting the required information" and second "utilizing the collected information". The process of collecting the required information is called as the "Case taking" and utilizing the collected information is known as "Case analysis". Both these steps must be performed in a precise orderly and artistic way if one wishes to get the expected result in each case.

A person who do not have any interest in drawing and if asked to draw an elephant then it would look like as shown below

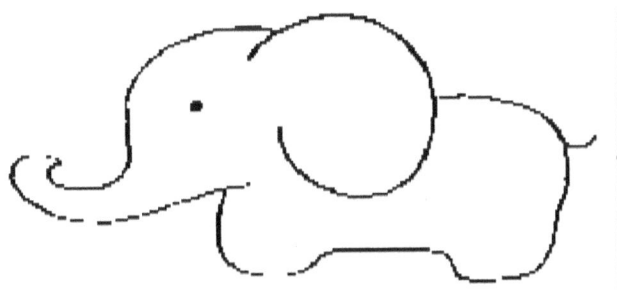

The above image although seems like an elephant is too far from being called as an artistic work. It is just a mechanical work which can be easily imitated by even someone who has the least interest in drawing.

Now have a look at the below image that resembles an artistic work

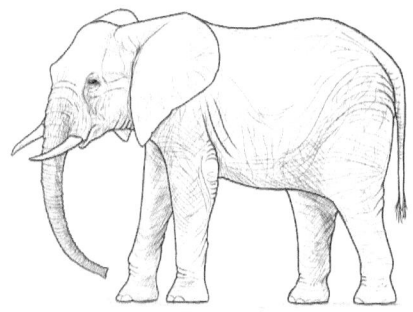

In order to perform the work in an artistic way you need interest, hard work, dedication, time and passion. These are the same requirements that one needs to possess to study and master this wonderful art of practicing classical homoeopathy.

We all know that Organon and Philosophy is the backbone based on which our entire system is built. Still, it's also a bitter truth that today majority of us have failed to comprehend it, resulting in the pathetic situation that we find ourselves today.

Now this gives rise to a very important question. If we all admit that "Organon and Philosophy" are the most subjects to learn why it is that majority of us have failed to comprehend it?

We do not need to go too far hunting for the answer as the answer is very clearly and very precisely mentioned in ur literature written years ago.

"Hahnemann's Organon is a strong, rich source of knowledge, but it is in long sentences, and very condensed, and difficult for many to understand."
(Lesser writings by J T Kent)

Organon is indeed a very rich source of knowledge but at the same time it is written in long sentences and goes difficult for many to understand. Now, when we fail to understand something then we are left with two options.

Option 1:

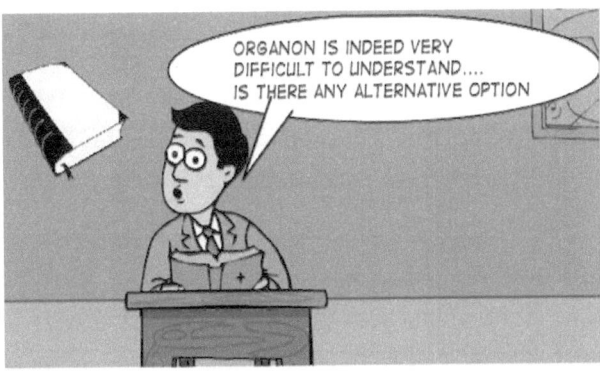

First option is to look for an alternative source to ensure self-survival by overlooking the organon and philosophy. When we decide to go with this option we are compromising. Compromising the patient's benefit, our own self earning and also with the growth of our entire system. Such people then tend to live their life in a survival mode where they have no concern for their own growth or for the growth of the system.

Option 2:

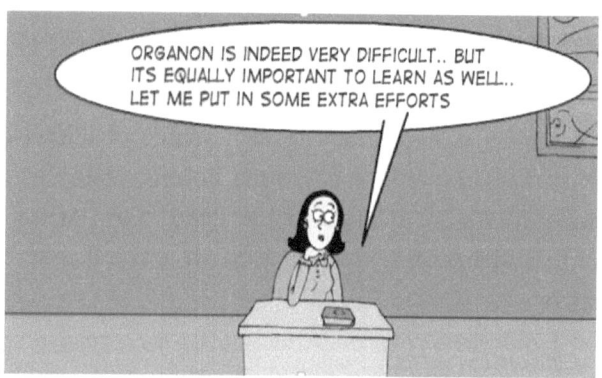

The second option is to realize the importance of understanding the 'Organon and Philosophy" and put some extra efforts to grasp and understand it.

The curiosity among such quality learner's shall definitely yield positive outcome when a little extra effort is put in and such people are the real assets to our entire homoeopathic fraternity and it's only because of such efforts our system has managed to survive till date despite facing heavy critics and serious allegations from those who pretend to own the monopoly over the profession of medical practice.

The second reason to account for the pathetic situation we are in today can again be quoted from our authentic literature

"Yet nearly all our colleges fail to teach these principles; the Chair of Philosophy may be filled by a man who knows nothing of the subject. Such a state of affairs delays the spread of Homoeopathy. Homoeopathy would develop faster if the physicians were all true to its principles. So many use the compound tablets, and prescribe tinctures in physiological doses, telling people they practice Homoeopathy" (Lesser writings by J T Kent)

Unfortunately if we correlate the existing scenario in the majority of colleges today with the above phrase it would not be a debatable point at all to admit that what has been mentioned in our authentic literature written years ago is nothing but a fact that holds true even today.

If the truth be told, the majority of us realize the need to understand the organon and philosophy only when we tend to get passed out and face the challenges in life to set up, run, maintain and flourish in our clinical practice. For many the pressure of survival and self earnings mounts to that extreme extent by then that they shall have no other option left but to look for their own existence and in such situations many often the interest of our patient and growth of our system becomes secondary.

"Conscience" is a person's moral sense of right and wrong, viewed as acting as a guide to one's behaviour.

Think about any favourite non-living asset that you own, be it your laptop, your desktop, your mobile or your vehicle. In a scenario when such a favourite thing of yours gets damaged and needs to be repaired will you ever hand it over to get it repaired to such a person whom you very well know that have no idea whatsoever as to how to repair it but is still trying to find a way out by trying his luck on your favourite thing?

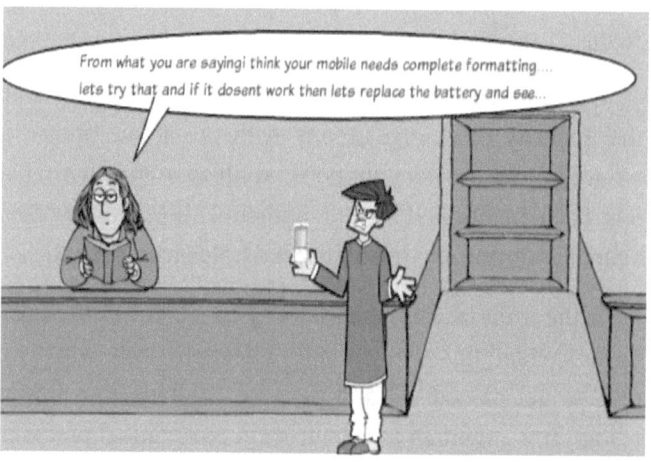

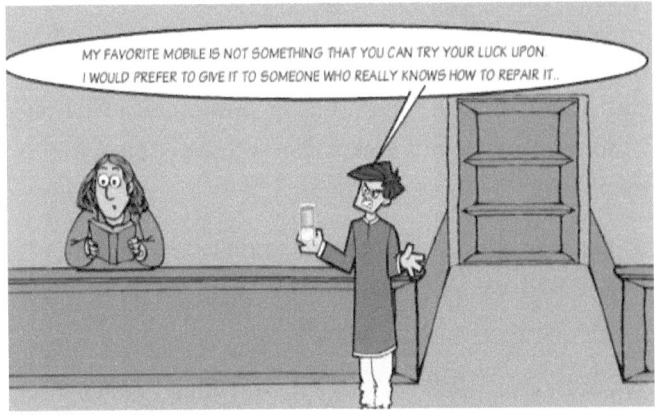

Now, it's quite an obvious reaction. We never would like to take chances with something that is important in our life. If this is the case then on what grounds we expect the people to come to us and also bring their loved ones to us for getting treated when from our conscience, we realize that we are also sitting setting up a clinic to try our luck upon our patients.

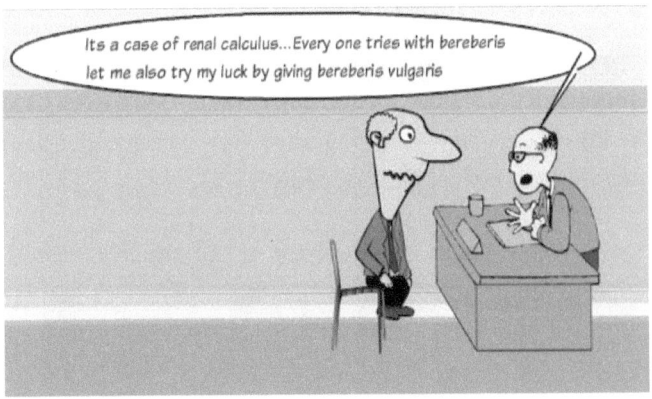

Just like we trust the person to whom we give our favourite asset to get it repaired, our patients too blindly trust us when they come to us or bring their loved ones to us under the impression that we are sitting here to treat them.

Isn't it then becomes our moral responsibility to ensure that we give our patients what he deserves the best to get from a homoeopath?

And can that best be anything under any circumstance less than a permanent cure in the shortest possible time?

Now, the question is how many of us are really capable of delivering the best possible output to our patients?

If majority were indeed capable of doing that then our system "Homoeopathy" would have been at a totally different level today. So, the fact shall have to be admitted that majority of us have failed to faithfully discharge our duty.

It is secondary to consider "what we know" but most importantly we first need to understand "What we need to know" if we wish to master this wonderful art of practicing classical homoeopathy.

So, let's begin this journey in an orderly way to explore this wonderful art of healing…...

1. Understanding the basics

Every science is governed by certain laws, theories and principles. Homoeopathy being a science is also built and laid upon certain laws, theories and principles. So, it becomes very essential for us to first understand these laws, theories and principles.

Planes of the body

Our body is made up of two planes. The outermost plane is called the materialistic plane while the innermost plane is called the dynamic plane.

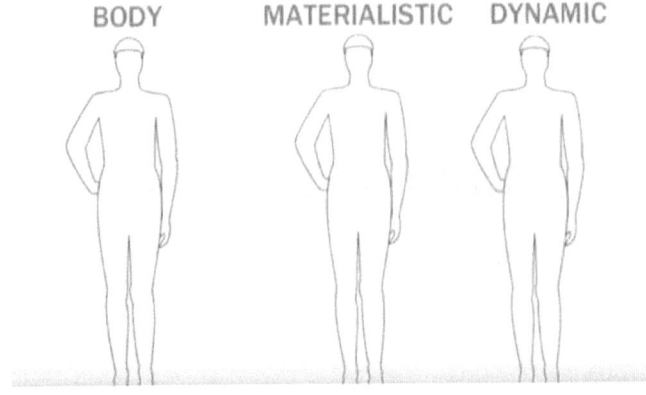

The outermost materialistic plane is composed of all the cells, tissues, organs, blood vessels and nerves.

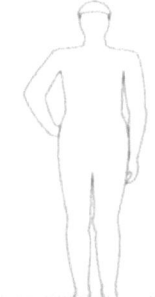

MATERIALISTIC PLANE

CELLS
TISSUES
ORGANS
BLOOD VESSELS
NERVES

The materialistic plane is under the control of the cerebellum, cerebrum ie the brain, spinal cord and nerves.

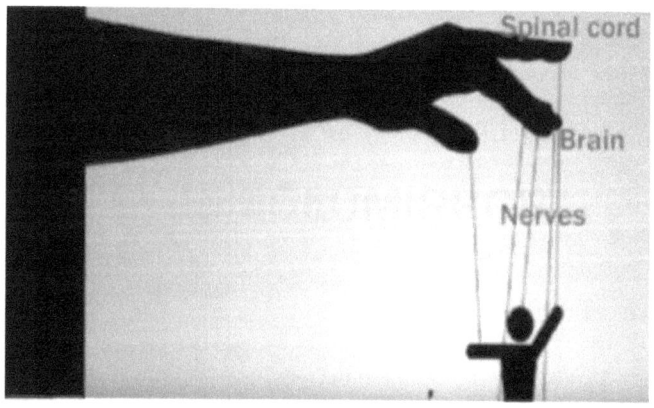

Skin forms a protective covering over the materialistic plane thereby protecting it from the external morbific disease causing agents.

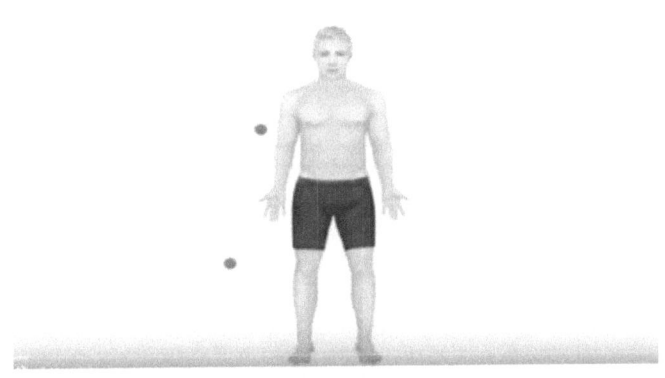

Deeper lies the dynamic plane which is composed of the VITAL FORCE acting as the central controlling unit, then our will and emotions and then our intellect and understanding.

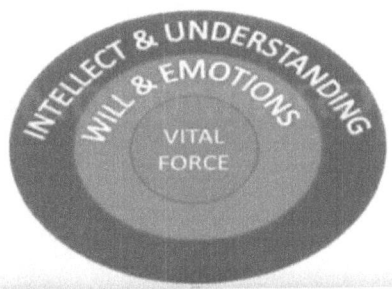

These two planes are interconnected with each other and neither of them can exist in isolation. This clearly means that when the vitality (dynamic plane) exhausts the material body also ceases to function (death). Similarly, extensive and irreparable damage to the materialistic body (for example in severe accidents) will automatically cause the vitality (dynamic plane) to sink and exhaust.

Both the dynamic and materialistic plane work in tandem ensuring that all the bodily functions are carried out smoothly and the person enjoys a feeling of being healthy both physically and mentally. If we can call the vital force as the central controlling unit then its activities is ensuring smooth functioning of all bodily activities, ensuring the person has no abnormal sensations, self protection and self preservation are executed and mediated at materialistic level by all the cells, tissues, organs, blood vessels and nerves under the control of the brain, spinal cord, and nerves.

Just like the skin forms a protective covering over the materialistic plane, the vital force also forms a protective covering at a dynamic level protecting the dynamic plane being acted upon by external negative dynamic influence

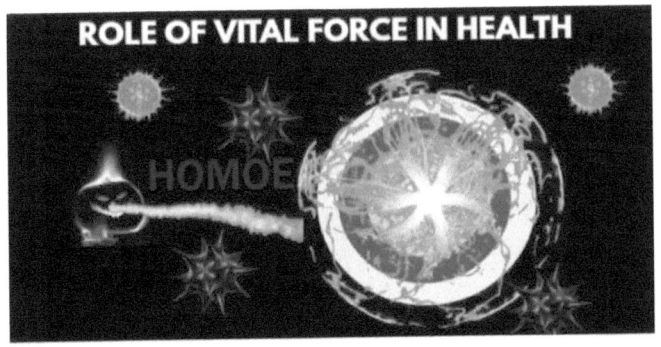

Dynamic Influence

Now, let's try to understand the meaning of dynamic influence. All those who believe in god when they go to temples, churches or any other religious places what do they get from there?

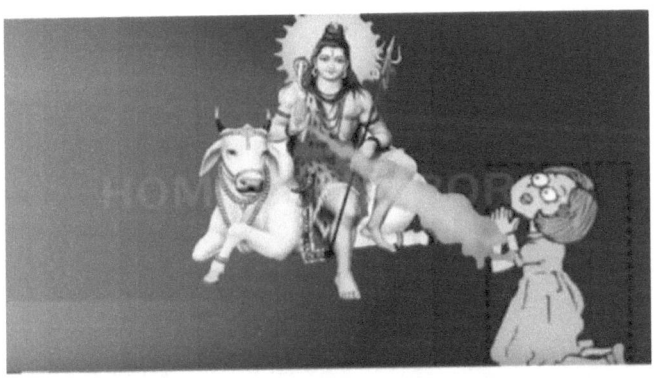

They acquire nothing but a "positive energy." Nowadays it's common to see a few people who call themselves as motivational speakers and when they deliver such motivational speeches, thousands of people go and attend it. These people also acquire nothing but a "positive energy" from the speaker. So basically, there are several sources from where such positive energy can be gained which includes

- *Motivation*
- *Prayers*
- *Meditation and Yoga*
- *Encouragement*
- *Success and pleasant news or incidents*
- *Hug or a simple smile*
- *Achievements etc*

Such positive energies always have a positive impact upon our body basically affecting the dynamic plane, but its positive effects get reflected through some positive changes even at materialistic level. (For example, positive energies leading to speedy recovery from diseases)

Now, to receive such positive energies one has to raise themselves dynamically to that level wherein they can acquire such positive energies. If one fails to raise themselves dynamically to the level where they can acquire this positive energy, then such energies shall have absolutely no effect upon him and it goes in vain. Let's try to understand these statements with some simple examples.

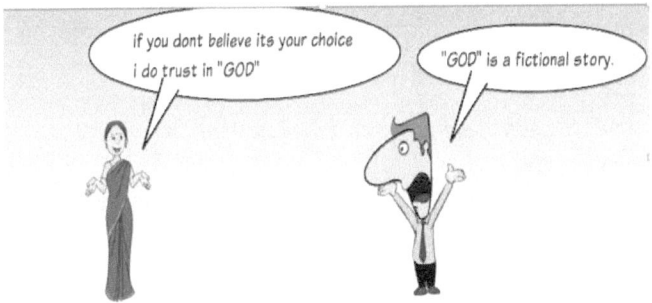

All those who do not believe in "God" they cannot acquire the positive energy from the religious places from where many others claim to have got benefited because their disbelief has not allowed to raise themselves dynamically to that level where they can acquire this positive energy.

Similarly, to get benefited from the positive energy emitted from any source, one has to first raise themselves dynamically to a level where they are in a position to acquire it.

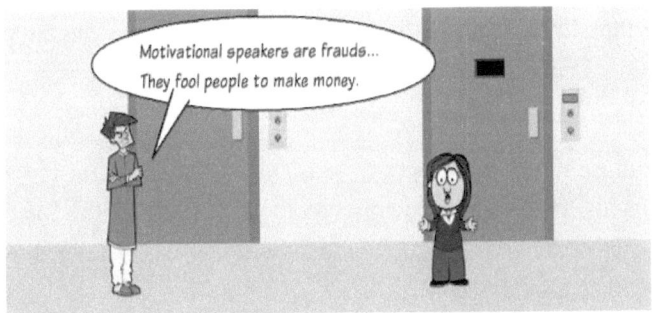

As we have discussed on positive energies there also exists something called the "negative energies". There are also various sources for this "negative energies" as well which includes

> *Demotivation and discouragement*
> *Sadness*
> *Depression*
> *Disappointment*
> *Failures*
> *Bad events and unpleasant incidents*
> *Grief and fear*
> *Anxiety, worry etc*

Both these positive and negative energy influences the body at a dynamic level and hence they are called "Positive dynamic influence" and "Negative dynamic influence" respectively.

Positive dynamic influence has a positive impact upon the body and plays a very important role in maintaining a person healthy and in curing him. On the other hand, negative dynamic influence has a negative impact upon the body and tends to make a person sick.

It is such negative dynamic influence existing in nature that tends to act dynamically upon the vital force trying to cause its derangement. When the vital force gets deranged by such negative dynamic influence it makes the person "Sick".

Effect of dynamic influence on Vital force

As we all know that the vital force is dynamic and spiritual in nature. So, if something has to have an effect upon it, then it should be also dynamic and spiritual in nature. The positive and negative dynamic influence has two contrasting influence upon the vital force. The positive dynamic influence has a positive effect upon the vital force and plays a very important role in maintating a state of health as well as in curing a person. It helps to strengthen the dynamic protective covering (see later) thereby preventing the negative dynamic influence to act upon the vital force.

Sometimes we observe that this overall positive state of mind protects the person from falling sick even after getting exposed to the exciting factors. Here is an example:

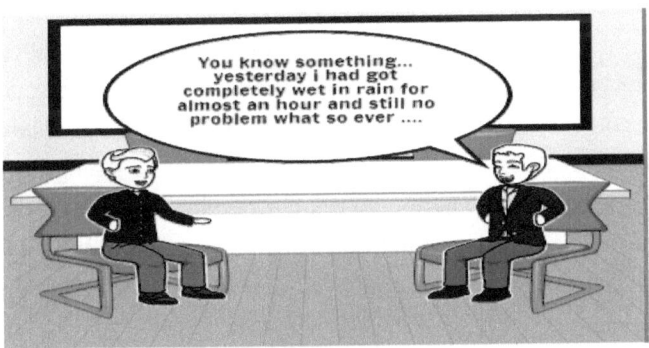

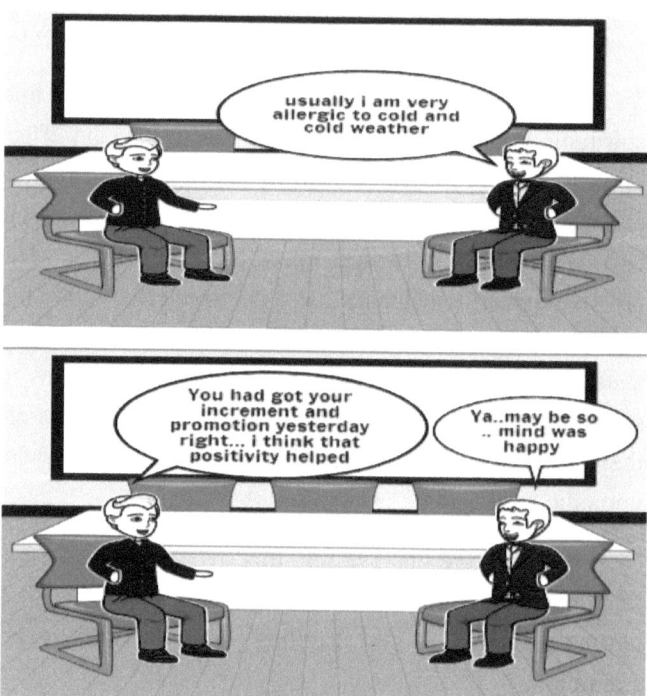

On the other hand, the negative dynamic influence has a negative impact upon both the strength of dynamic protective covering as well as on the vital force. They tend to make a person sick by lowering the strength of dynamic protective covering thereby allowing the external negative dynamic influence to act upon the vital force threatening to cause its derangement. Here is an example:

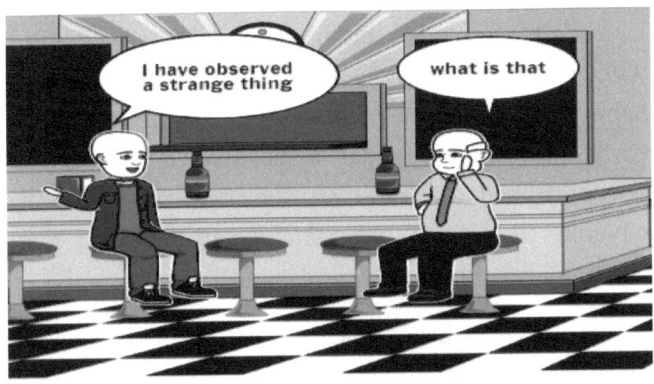
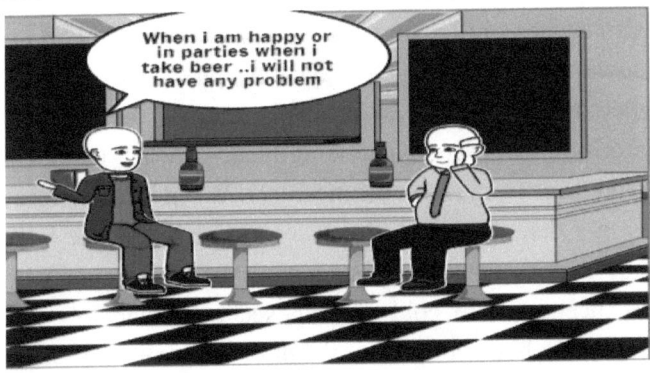
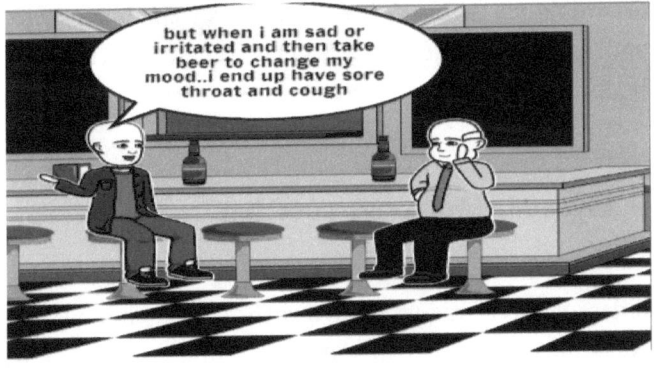

Let's try to explain the above findings co-relating it with what we had discussed above. When someone is happy (happiness is a positive influence) or enjoying in parties (enjoyment again a positive influence) this positivity adds strength to the dynamic protective covering keeping it intact and keeps the vital force protected from the negative dynamic influence.

On the other hand, when the person is sad (sadness negative dynamic influence) or depressed (depression is also negative influence) this sadness or depression brings down the strength of the dynamic protective covering thereby making it weak. This allows the external morbific negative dynamic influence to act upon the vital force to cause its derangement. When the vital force is in a deranged state it exposes the body and the body becomes suceptabile. In such a condition someone who is suceptabile to cold get exposed to it tend to cause problems like sore throat, cough or any other complaint according his own suceptability. The suceptability factor and its role in disease has been discussed later in this book.

Dynamic protective covering

From the above discussion we have seen clearly that unless the dynamic protective covering does not become weak the external negative dynamic influence cannot act upon the vital force to cause its derangement. So basically, a person falls sick only when the dynamic protective covering has weakened. This clearly means that there are certain factors upon which the strength of this dynamic protective covering depends upon the factors which lower the strength of dynamic protective covering can be broadly divided into two types.

a. External
b. Internal

External factors are those which have an impact from outside. This includes

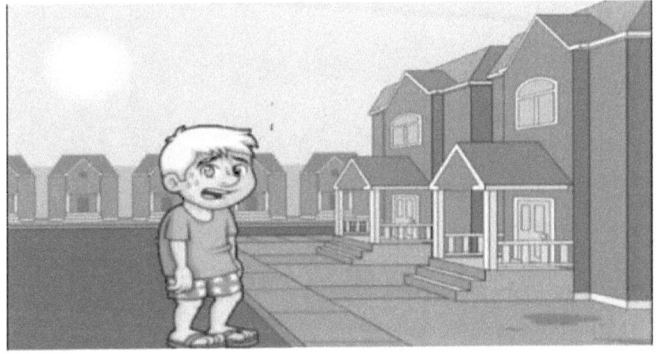

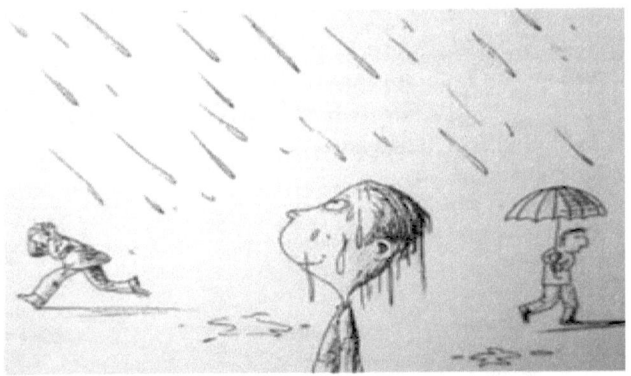

Getting exposed to extreme climatic conditions

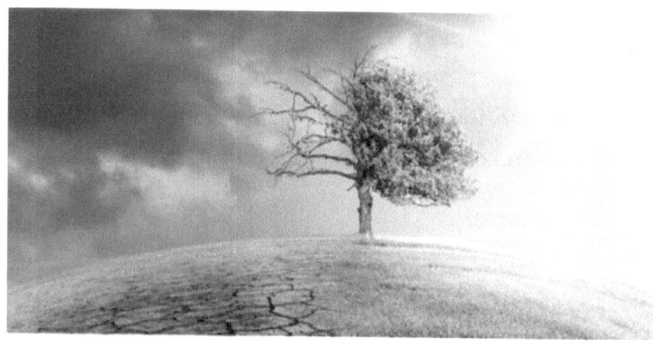

Sudden chage in external atmosphere

Internal factors can further be divided into two categories

a. Mental
b. Physical

Mental factors include

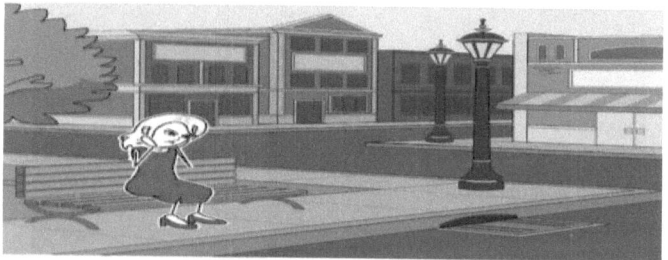

Sadness, depression & disappointments

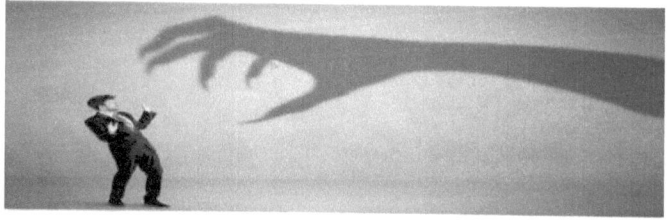

Fear & Fright

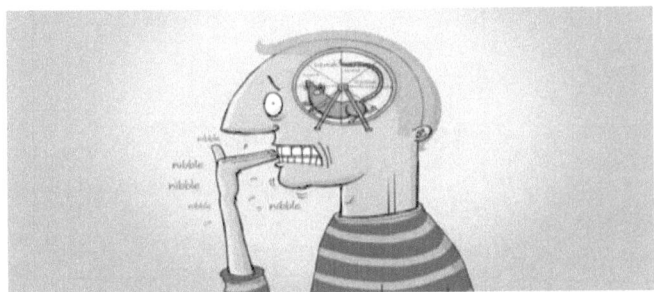

Anxiety, tension & Panic

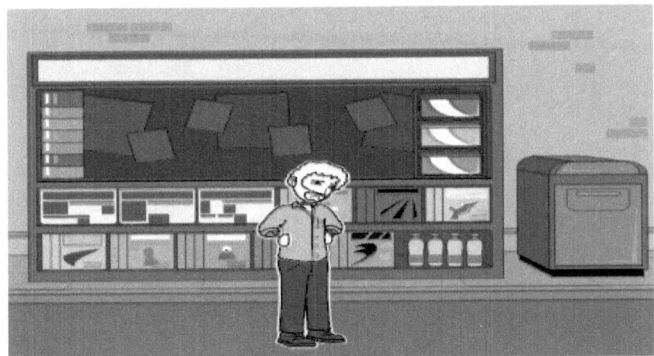

Failures & Bad news

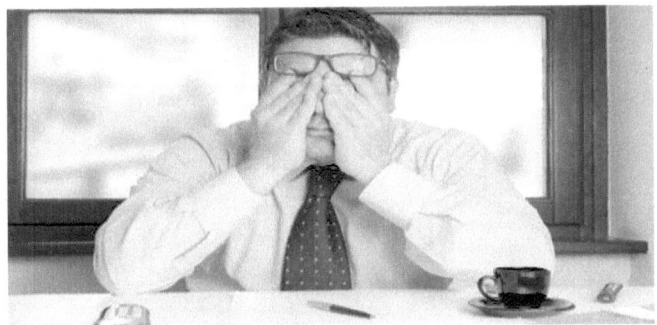

Over mental exertion, exhaustion & strain

Physical factors include:

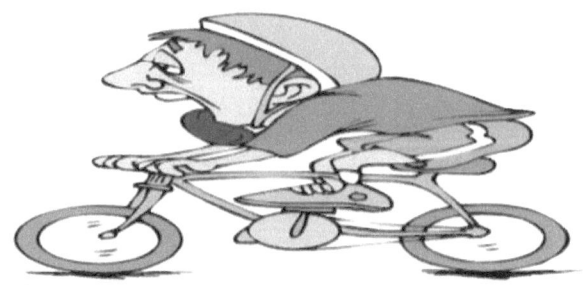

Over or unusual physical exertion

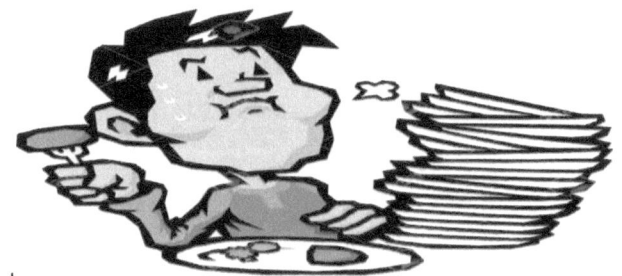

Overeating

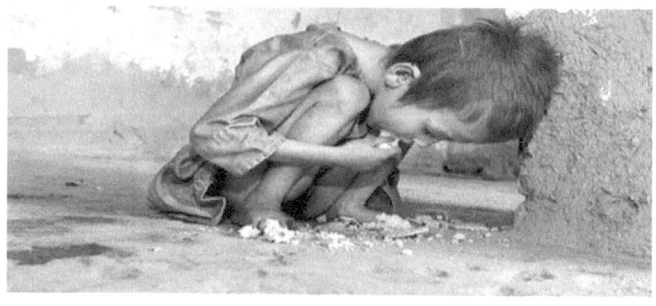

Starving or malnutrition

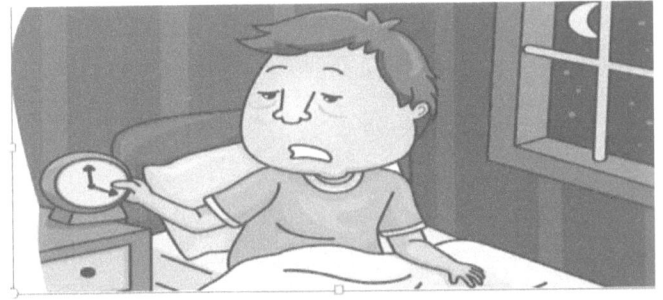

Sleeplessness

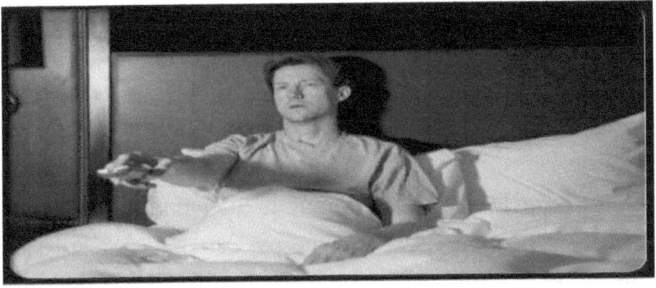

Night watching

In short, all those factors which can disturb the internal harmony both at mental and physical plane can result in lowering of the strength of the dynamic protective covering.

It also must be remembered that these factors discussed above shall not unconditionally have the same effect in each and every individual. The overall impact and extent of damage done shall depend on various factors taken together both at mental and physical plane. Let's consider an example to understand this in a better way. Have a look at the two images given below

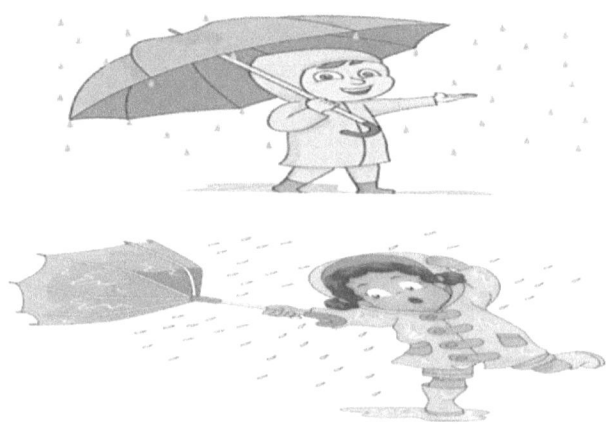

Now as you can see in the first image the affected person is enjoying the condition and in such a situation chances of lowering the strength of dynamic protective covering becomes less and the person shall not fall sick provided his physical body is not too weak to induce sickness.

On the other hand, in the second image the affected person is not enjoying the condition he is in and in such a situation the chances are high that the strength of the dynamic protective layer shall be lowered, and the person may fall sick.

So, all these factors discussed above work in tandem to decide the final outcome. This is the reason why all those people who get exposed to the same exciting factors do not fall sick.

Similarly, the factors which give strength to the dynamic protective covering can also be divided broadly into two categories

1. *External*
2. *Internal*

These factors include sources from where positive energy can be acquired. This includes

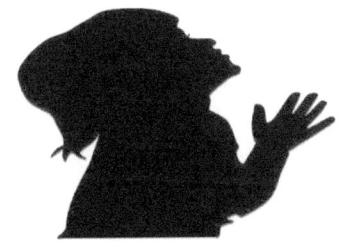

Prayers

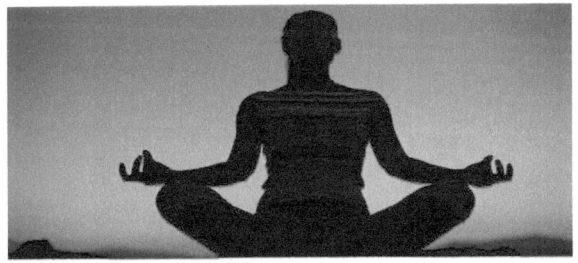

Meditation & yoga

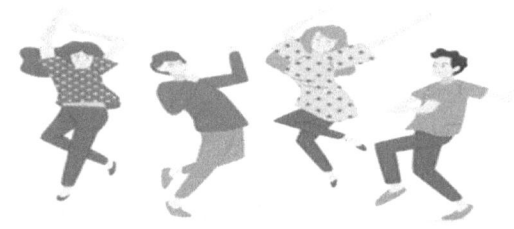

Enjoyment & entertainment

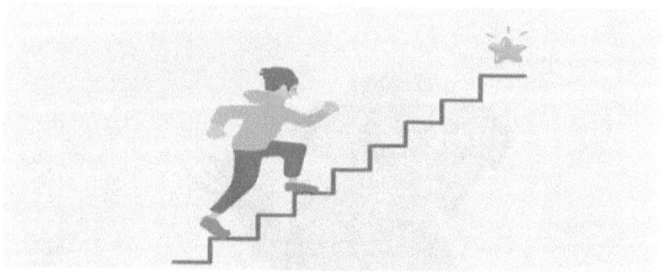

Success & achievements

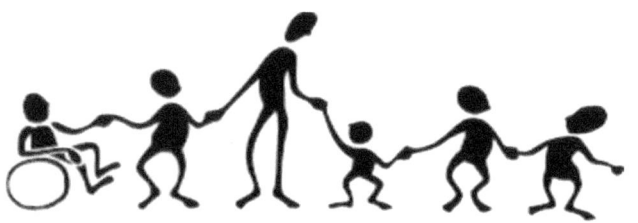

Caring & love

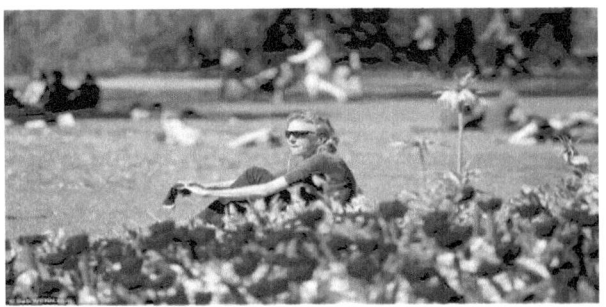

Favorable environmental conditions

On one hand the factors that tend to bring down the strength of the dynamic protective covering contributes towards making a person sick, on the other hand the factors that help to strengthen the dynamic protective covering helps the person to maintain a state of health and also plays an important role in his recovery. The vital force when in order ensures that the strength of this protective dynamic covering is maintained so that the external negative dynamic influence is not allowed to act upon the vital force.

Role of vital force in health

" The material organism, without the vital force, is capable of no sensation, no function, no self-preservation, it derives all sensation and performs all the functions of life solely by means of the immaterial being (the vital principle) which animates the material organism in health and in disease" (Aphorism 10)

It becomes very clear from the above aphorism that the materialistic plane without the vital force is capable of no sensation, no function, no self preservation. Its is the vital force which ensures the smooth functioning of all the bodily activities. It is also responsible for the self preservation. When we talk about self preservation two aspects needs to be discussed. One is to protect the thing which needs self preservation from anything that can cause a threat to cause damage or destruction and second ensure that such threats are eliminated or removed on time even before they can cause damage or destruction.

Vital force when in order ensures and serves to achieve both the above discussed objectives of self preservation. It forms the protective covering at a dynamic level (see below fig) thereby not allowing the external negative dynamic influence to act upon the vital force and cause its derangement. It also ensures that any threat (in the form of any morbific agents) if gained entry into the body is eliminated or removed on time even before they can cause any possible destruction or damage. This function is mediated at materialistic level through the defense mechanisms which includes the role of RBC's, WBC's and platelets

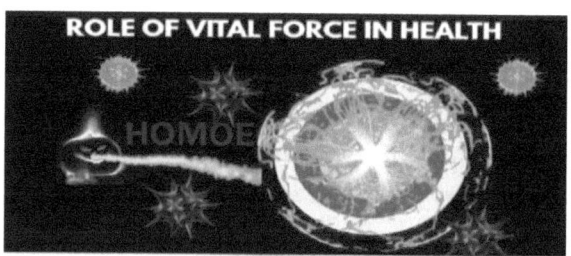

What makes a person sick?

In the last chapter we had discussed as to how the dynamic protective covering protects the vital force from being acted upon by negative dynamic influence and when this protective covering becomes weak the vital force is acted upon by the negative dynamic influence that tends to cause its derangement

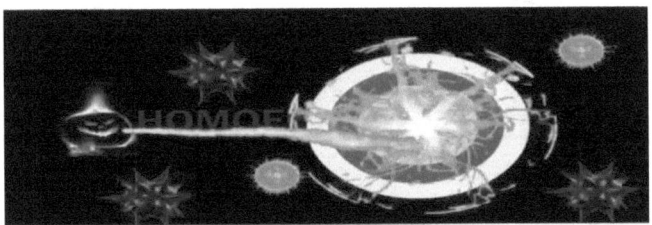

This derangement creates an imbalance and this imbalance shall flow from the centre to the periphery affecting first our will and emotions then our intellect and understanding, then the physical generalities are altered and finally the physical symptoms appear.

Hence the alterations are found at general level much before the physical symptoms appear. (See examples below)

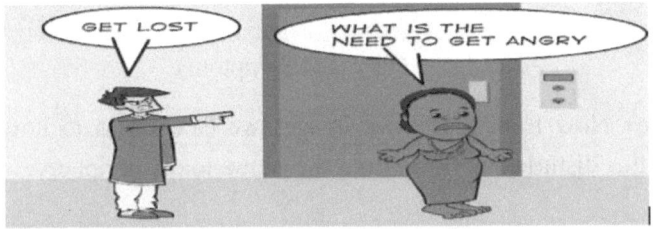

Unusual anger (Emotional level symptom)

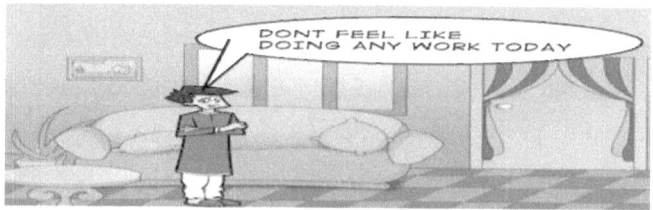

Indolence or laziness (Intellectual level symptom)

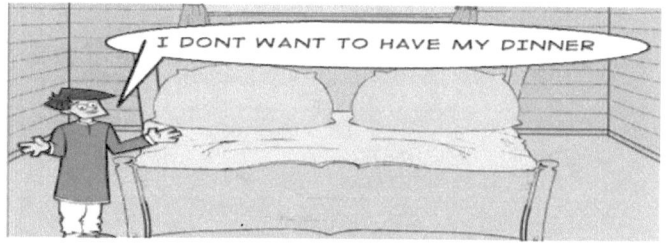

Loss of appetite (Altered physical general)

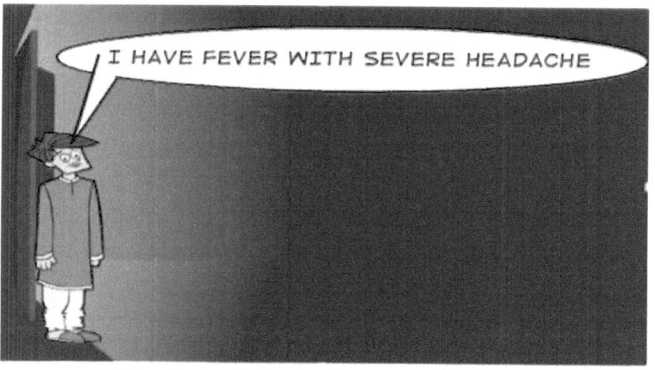

Headache (Physical Symptom)

Now from the above images we can see as to how this disturbance flows from the centre to the periphery.

Let's try to understand this with a simple example. Look at the water in the below image. It's still and steady.

Now let's see as to what happens when a drop of water falls into this container.

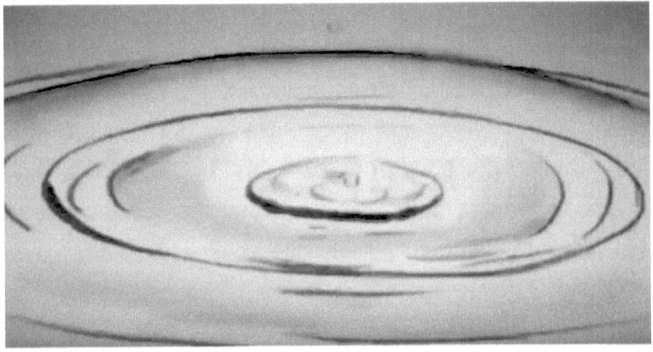

As you can see above the water drop created a disturbance and this disturbance flowed in the form of waves from the centre where it was created outwardly to the periphery.

Similarly, when the vital force gets deranged the disturbance thus created shall also flow from the centre to the periphery affecting first the mental plane and then the physical plane finally getting settled at one or more localized parts over the physical plane.

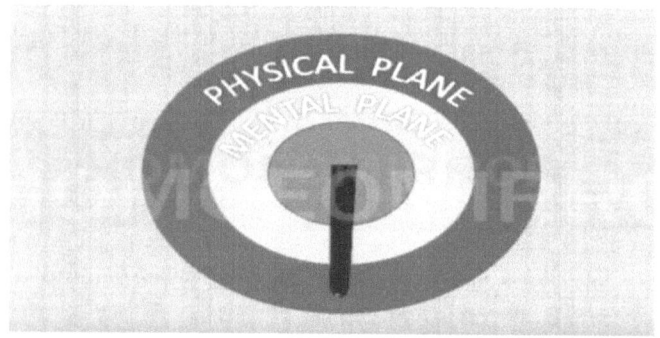

Now if for instance this disturbance gets localized in lungs that part becomes more prone to develop physical symptoms and shall provide a soil for the growth and multiplication of pathogens and microbes giving rise to yet another group of symptoms. Such symptoms when grouped together gives it a name which we call as the "clinical diagnosis". In this case we may name it as lung fibrosis, Asthma, bronchitis, Tuberculosis etc depending on what kind of physical symptoms are produced and we attribute the blame to the poor pathogens that the microscope or culture can trace. (For example, Mycobacterium Tubeculi receives the blame for causing Tuberculosis).

Disease ultimates

So, these set of physical symptoms that appear are in fact not the beginning, but they are the endings. They are not diseases, but they are called the "Disease Ultimates". In homoeopathy we treat the disease and not the disease ultimates. All the diagnostic names that we give to a set of common symptoms be it asthma, arthritis, migraine, hepatitis, fibrosis etc are nothing but the disease ultimates.

Let's see some references from our literature that explains the same as what we have discussed above.

"To heal the sick, man must perceive what in the body is in disorder, and he can perceive this only by viewing the phenomena of disorder.

The phenomena that represent progress from cause to effect are often ignored until ultimates that can be seen and touched are present. This assumes that a thing can be a thing and at the same time the cause of itself." (Lesser writings J T Kent)

"The laboratory conducts study not of life, nor of disease, but of results of disease. That causes are sometimes continued into effects is true, but knowledge of the endings of causes is useless except in relation to knowledge of their beginnings and the course by which they develop". (Lesser writings J T Kent)

> *"It must now be seen that the physician who has in mind only the pathology as a basis for his prescription has only what is most common, and therefore has no view of the totality, and therefore violates the first principles of prescribing. He prescribes for results, for endings, and not for things first, not for causes." (Lesser writings J T Kent)*

> *"It must be understood, however, that the diagnosis does not reveal the nature of a disease in a manner to image a remedy. The diagnosis is the name of ultimates and exteriors, while it is, the interior nature that must be perceived through the peculiar, characterizing signs and symptoms, in order to discover the remedy that will cure." (Organon §§ 6-8.). (Lesser writings J T Kent)*

It's very evident from what has been quoted above that in the hunt for reaching at the right similimum the symptoms of disease ultimates have least role to patient. So how fair it is to then list remedies for various clinical conditions like best remedies for asthma, arthritis, migraine or hepatitis?

Role of vital force in disease

In a state of disease, the normal functioning of the body or the part affected is in a compromised state or shows abnormal physical symptoms. The vital foce being in a disordered state cannot perform the function of protection and self preservation. Hence in such a state it is incapable of removing the physical symptoms.

Source of physical symptoms

The derangement of vital force alone does not result in producing physical symptoms, but it only triggers abnormal sensations and functions at a general level as the disturbance flows from the centre to the periphery. When this disturbance gets localized on the materialistic plane at one or more parts, these parts becomes susceptible and provides a platform or soil for the growth of morbific agents like bacterias, viruses and other pathogens. In cases where no external morbific agents are involved (like simple headache) the disturbance thus localized makes that part susceptible to produce physical symptoms.

Let's consider an example to make this clearer.

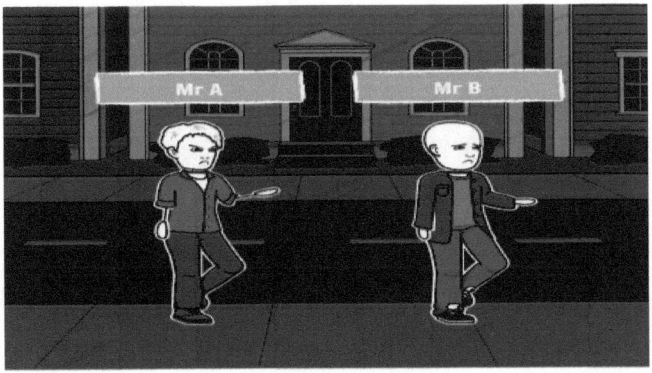

In the above example two persons Mr A and Mr B got wet in an unexpected rain that came suddenly. This trigerring factor lowered the strength of the dynamic protective covering followed by which the negative dynamic influence acted upon the vital force causing its derangement. This derangement creates and imbalance which then flows from the centre to the periphery affecting first the will and emotions then the intellect and understanding are affected, then the physical generalities are altered and finally this disturbance shall get settled locally on the materialistic plane in one or more parts. Before this disturbance reaches the materialistic plane let's compare the changes observed in both Mr A and Mr B

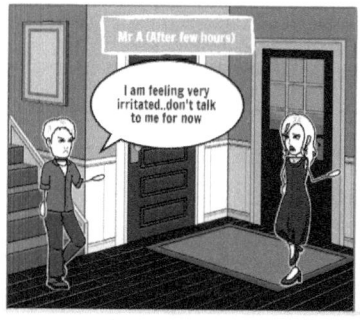
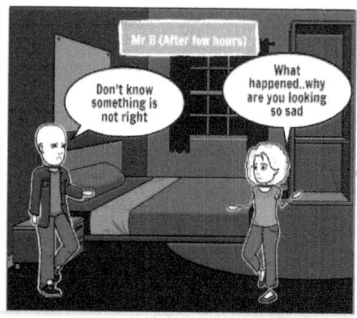
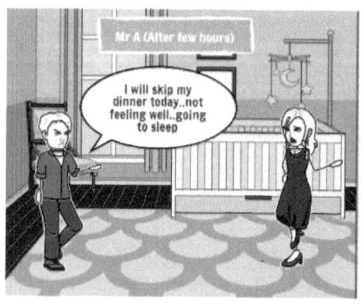
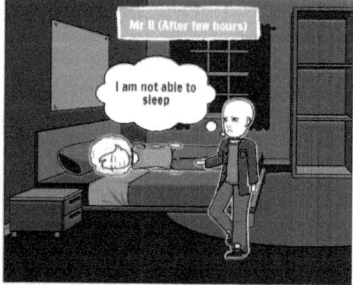

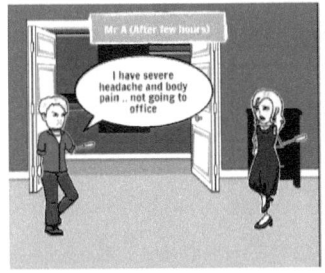 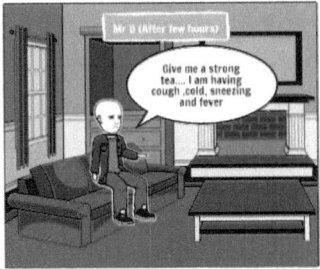

As you can notice both for Mr A and Mr B the factor trigerring the disturbance was same ie getting wet in rain. But Mr A developed irritation (alteration at mental level) followed by loss of appetite (altered physical general) and finally ended up in having body ache and headache (disease ultimate).

For Mr B it started with feeling of sadness (altered mental symptom) followed by sleeplessness (altered physical general) and finally ended up in having cough, cold coryza, sneezing and fever (disease ultimates). So, depending upon in which part the disturbance shall get localized accordingly physical symptoms developed shall vary. This varation will be different in different people and also it may differ in the same person in different situations (will be discussed later in detail).

When the vital force is deranged the imbalance thus created when flows from centre to periphery as it affects the mental plane first there shall be a response or reaction at individual level which is felt or get reflected as the mental symptoms of altered disposition.

Similarly, when this imbalance affects the physical plane then also there shall be such an individualistic reaction or response which then constitutes towards the alteration in physical generalities and at localized level it gives rise to the characteristic particulars and concomitants.

It must be therefore very clearly understood that aleered mental symptoms, altered physical generals, characteristic particulars and concomitants are not related to the disease ultimates of the patient but they represent the individualstic reaction or response to the flow of imbalance. Hence this group of symptoms has to be collected from each and every case to construct the totality of the case.

Sick

"The physician's high and only mission is to restore the sick to health, to cure, as it is termed (Aphorisim 1)"

From this first aphorism we should clearly try to perceive the meaning of the term "Sick". As we have already discussed when the dynamic protective covering becomes weak the vital force is acted upon by external negative dynamic influence causing its derangement. Vital force in such a deranged state fails to accomplish its role of protection and self preservation. As a result a person experiences abnormal sensations and functions. These alterations occur much prior to the appearance of physical symptoms over the materialistic plane. In such a state where the vital force is in a deranged state and its functions are compromised, we call the person to be

"Sick". Sickness is a term related to the person as a whole and is not being referred to any physical symptoms appearing in any localized part of the body.

It's said that in Homeopathy we treat the patient and not his disease. This clearly means that we need to consider the patient as a whole. Many a times you may come across patient's who will have plenty of complaints to narrate. They shall enumerate pages of symptoms, pages of sufferings, they look sick and they themselves have a strong feeling that they are not well but despite consulting the specialists and conducting all possible examinations and tests the specialists may fail to trace anything abnormal from his physical body to declare him as "Sick". For them a person can be declared as being "Sick" if they have something abnormal to trace at materialistic level.

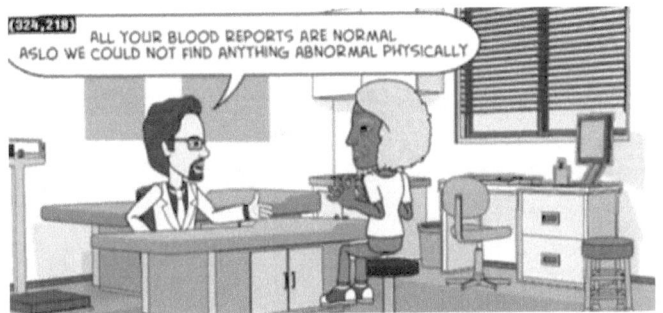

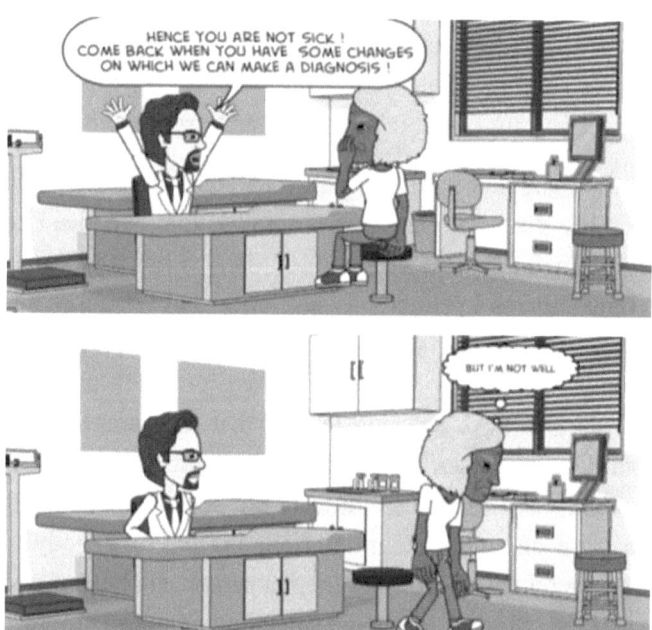

In such situations they prefer to wait until the physical symptoms appear and in some cases by then it would have become too late for the changes to get reversed.

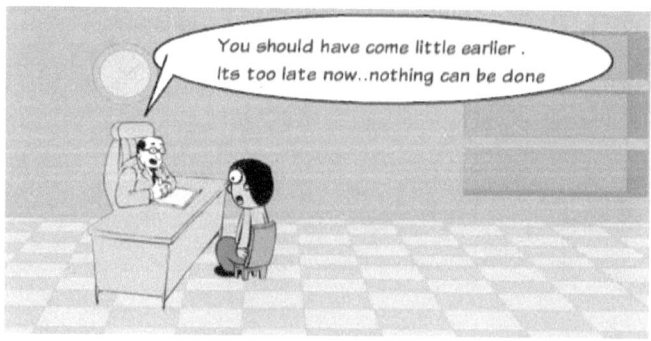

If somebody is having liver cirrhosis it has to be understood that he is sick, so he is having liver cirrhosis and not the other way around. It's the person who is sick as a whole and not just his liver. In such cases if it's only considered that his liver is sick and treated accordingly then the chances are there that the same person shall either have a relapse of his complaints at the same location or shall have some other organ affected sooner or later. People treated in such a way mostly keep on roaming from one specialty clinic to the other for years together.

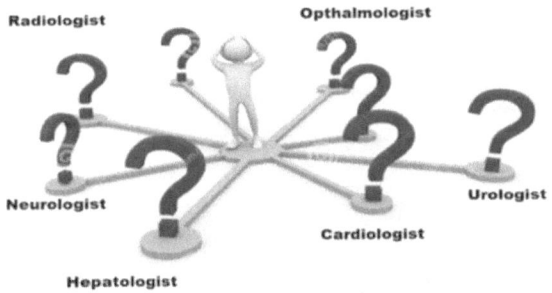

It's very important for us to understand that it's the person who becomes sick and not his organs or parts. The early signs of alterations both at mental level (both emotional and intellectual) and physical level indicates that the person is "Sick" and needs to be treated.

Step by step approach to practice classical homoeopathy

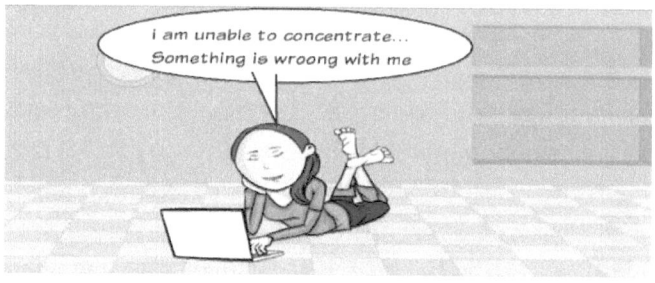

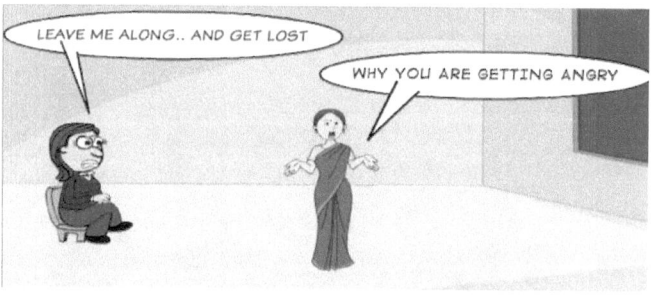

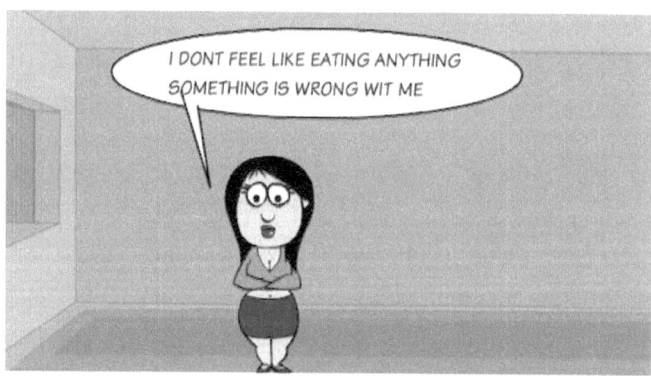

These individual symptoms are the only true guide that shall help us in the hunt for reaching at the right similimum.

What to expect from our remedies and where it acts?

We have already discussed that as given in the 10th aphorism of organon (6th edition) the vital force when in order is responsible for protection, self preservation and also to ensure that all the bodily activities are carried on smoothly. When the vital force gets deranged it then fails to perform these functions.

It must be kept in mind that a person suffers from disease producing thus producing physical or experiences abnormal sensations and functions only because the vital force is not in order. These physical symptoms or abnormal sensations and functions shall disappear automatically once the vital force is restored back to order because then the vital force which is now in order shall ensure the smooth functioning, protection and self preservation of the body. Our well selected remedies acts only upon the vital force to help it restore back to order. Those who believe that they are directing our remedies against any germs, worms or tumours that the patient may be having, is in extreme darkness for the simple reason that if the body was healthy and vital force was in order it would not have provided a soil favouring the growth of these germs, worms or tumors. Here is the reference for this from the lesser writings by J T Kent

"The man who believes that he is directing his remedies against germs, or against worms, or against a tumor the patient may have, is in extreme darkness, if he

cannot perceive that a healthy man will have healthy tissue, healthy blood, and therefore there can be no soil for germs and worms or morbid growths. (§§ 7, 11, 12, 14, 70, 84, 89, 98, 107-9.)"

2. Studying a drug from materia medica

When books tell you that drug is good for this or that pay no attention to them, but when book tells you that a drug has produced such and such symptoms study these; that is a piece of valuable information. J.T. Kent

It's very clear from the above phrase that there is no point in remembering that a drug is good for this or that, but it must be studied and understood as to what are the symptoms a drug has produced. This means that every symptom produced by a drug must be studied with respect to its various possibilities of getting observed in our clinical practice.

As we have seen above that every drug can reflect multiple conceptual images which is beyond the capability of human brain to remember. Hence while making an attempt to study a drug from the materia medica it has to be given more importance to understand these various conceptual images reflected by a remedy so that it can be easily compared with the image of sickness thereby helping us to find out the right similimum for the given case.

Some of us also have the habit of memorizing a few keynotes from each drug and we base our prescriptions on the basis of this memorized fragments of information given under a drug. As Dr Kent has said *"A keynote prescriber is but a memory prescriber; he has memorized only and has not made it a part of his understanding."*

In Homeopathy there are no surogates

Hahnemann has said that in Homeopathy there are no surrogates. Surrogates mean a substitute. This clearly means that for a given case although there can be a number of remedies running close to be the similimum the perfect similimum can be only one and no other remedy can do what that perfect similimum can.

As we have seen earlier that a single remedy can reflect multiple conceptual images but a person who is sick can have only one such image i.e., the image of sickness or portrait of disease. This image or portrait has to be exactly fit in with one of such multiple images reflected by a remedy. That remedy then becomes the perfect similimum for the given case.

So, the real task involves in learning how to construct the image of sickness perfectly and then to perfectly match with the image reflected by the remedy. From this its very clear that the remedy cannot be decided for a given case without forming the image of sickness and this image of sickness can be only constructed precisely when we have a complete case in hand.

When we say that for a given case the perfect similimum can be only one then it means that if multiple people are allowed to work on the same case individually at the end they all should come up with the same remedy as their indicated one. But clinically is it possible?

If it's not possible clinically then was our master Hahnemann wrong? when he made a statement that in homeopathy there can be no surrogates or is it that we go wrong somewhere?

Let's try to understand this with the help of a simple activity. Have a look at the image. It shows a number of Indian currency notes of various denominations.

Step by step approach to practice classical homoeopathy

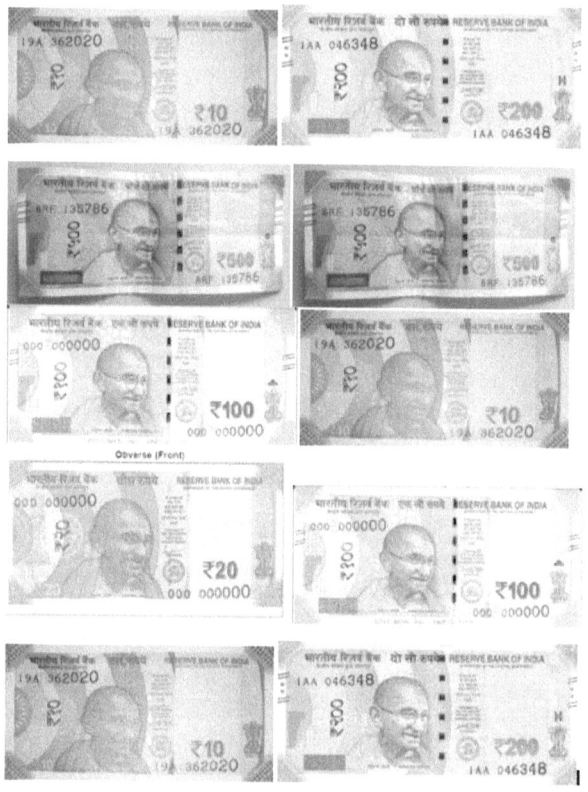

Now as you can see in the above image that there are two notes each having denominations of 100, 200 and 500 rupees respectively. Three notes of 10 rupees denomination and one note having Rupees 20 denomination.

Now if you are asked to pick out any 5 notes from the above combinations then you shall certainly pick up 2 notes having 500 denominations first , then 2 notes having 200 denominations and 1 note have 100 denominations. You shall never bother to even consider the notes having lesser values.

But if we ask a 4-year-old child to do this same activity then he shall randomly pick up any 5 notes as he wishes without bothering to consider it's value.

What made the difference here?

Since you knew the value of each of these notes you opted to pick up only those notes which were having higher values whereas a 4 year old child who does not know the value of these notes shall end up in picking any 5 notes randomly.

If these notes can be compared with the observed symptoms in a case then just like each note has its own value and importance similarly each of the observed symptoms in a case has got its own value and if one knows to give appropriate value to an observed symptom then while forming the totality and constructing the image of sickness he shall consider only those symptoms which is having the highest value.

Also if we all are perfect in our case taking art then even if hundred people work out on the same case individually they shall all have more or less the same symptoms to work with, although some may be able to trace few additional symptoms whereas some may miss out a few but no one shall ever miss out on any important symptoms from the given case.

This means that while analyzing the symptoms almost everyone will have more or less the same symptoms included in their totality thereby reaching at almost the same conceptual image of sickness and post repertorization each and every one shall reach at the same remedy as the indicated one.

This justifies the statement given by our master that in homoeopathy there are no surrogates. So, which means that majority of us go wrong somewhere but the question here to ask is where do we tend to go wrong?

We may go wrong at two places. One, we go wrong in taking the case completely so that we miss out to collect or observe important symptoms. Secondly, we do not know as to how to give proper value to an observed symptom. When we go wrong in giving value to an observed symptom, we shall end up in picking up wrong symptoms while constructing our totality which then shall yield an imperfect conceptual image leading to selection of a wrong remedy.

Conceptual image of remedy

There are hundreds of symptoms recorded and listed in our materia medica under each drug. The main source of this information recorded has come from the drug proving. But again, it doesn't mean that all the listed and recorded symptoms under a drug were unconditionally observed in all the provers. When the recorded symptoms under a drug are logically arranged it also then reflects an image which is termed as the "Conceptual image of the remedy".

Have a look at the word given below:

DOG

As we read this word "dog" the image of a dog immediately flashes in our mind at least for a second. But if we reverse the alphabets and then read, the meaning now changes completely also the image that will flash in our minds shall also change because when these letters are reversed it then becomes "GOD".

GOD

As we have just seen when the same letters are logically rearranged everytime it gives a new meaning and shall reflect a new image. Similarly, if these letters can be compared with the recorded symptoms of a drug, the logical re-arrangement of these symptoms shall reflect a new image each and every time. This means that every remedy can reflect such "N" number of conceptual images based on how the symptoms are rearranged.

Generally, majority of us have a tendency to memorize and remember a few symptoms from each drug and when we do not observe those in our patient, we tend to overlook that remedy. This is where we go wrong because remedy is not selected based on the few keynote symptoms observed but the overall image reflected in a sick person must fit in with the conceptual image reflected by a remedy.

This also explains as to how the same remedy can fit in as the similimum for different patients having different symptoms.

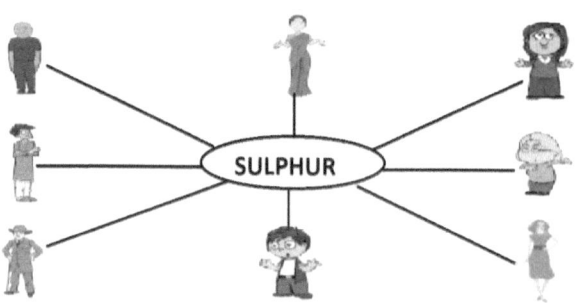

Image of sickness or portrait of disease

Have a look at the group of alphabets randomly arranged. These alphabets when joined randomly (as shown below) do not form a word that has a valid meaning.

| WORBENIGLTA |

Now, let's try to rearrange some of the above letters to form a meaningful word that represents the name of an animal or a bird.

| WORBENIGLTA |

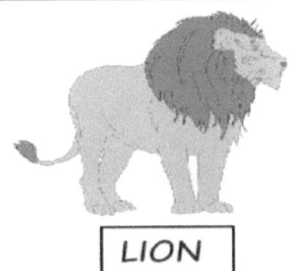

| LION |

WORBENIGLTA

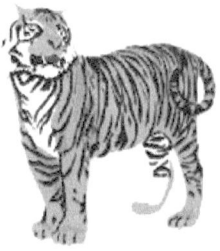

TIGER

WORBENIGLTA

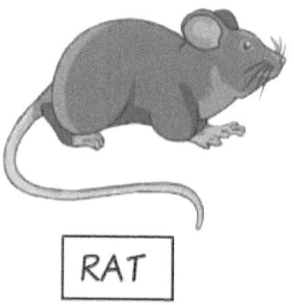

RAT

WORBENIGLTA

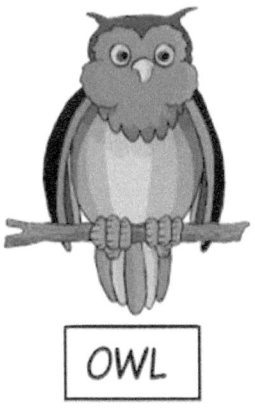

OWL

As you can see above when the same set of given letters were logically rearranged to form the name of an animal or a bird, we could form lion, tiger, rat, owl etc. Each of these animals has their own identity and image which immediately flashes in our mind the moment we spell or write that individual word.

Now let's compare the letters as the symptoms observed in a case and when we logically rearrange few of them based on their importance such logical arrangement shall also reflect an image. This image is called the image of sickness or portrait of the disease or conceptual image of sickness. So, this means that when we combine and logically rearrange the qualified symptoms out of a case in an orderly way the totality thus constructed reflects the image of sickness or portrait of the disease. The very purpose of taking a case in detail is to construct a totality to form the image of sickness or portrait of the disease.

Individualization

"Every remedy has in itself a certain state of peculiarities that identifies it as an individualremedy, and the patienthas also a certain state of peculiarities that identifies him as anindividual patient, and so the remedy is fitted to the patient." (J T kent)

In Homoeopathy its said that we treat a patient and not his disease. In earlier section we had seen that it's the patient who becomes sick and not his individual parts or organs and hence it's the patient who has to be treated as a whole, not his individual part or organs.

It must be kept in mind that no two individuals can be alike. Even in case of identical twins who appear to be alike in their physical appearance there shall still be a lot of individual pecularities in them that help to differentiate between the two individuals.

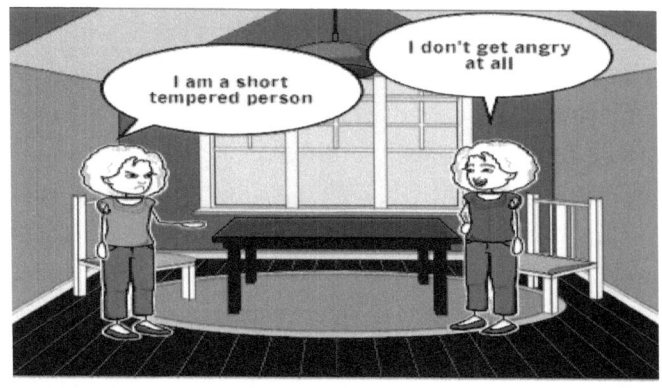
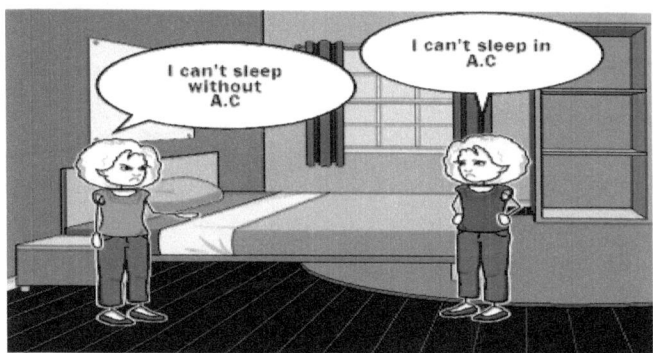
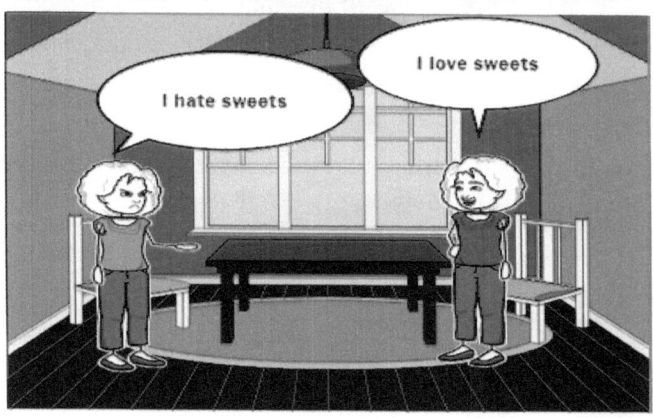

There are such set of individual pecularities or characters in each and every individual both in their state of health and the way they react towards a disturbance. These pecularities helps to differentiate one person from the other even though both may be having the same diease. Such set of individual symptoms or pecularities when grouped together forms the individualizing symptoms of the person and this process is known as "Individualization".

Individulaization plays a key role in guiding towards the right similimum for a given case. A remedy which may have worked for an individual having let's say bronchial asthma shall not work in each and every person having broncial asthma because the remedy is selected on the basis of this individualizing pecularities that can never be exactly the same in two different individuals.

It must be remembered that individualization is done on the basis of the symptoms or pecularities that belong to the person and not on the basis of the common symptoms of the disease. For the same reason in Homeopathy the remedies cannot be listed on the basis of the disease ultimates or clinical diagnosis.

Perfect Similimum

As already discussed in the other section in Homoeopathy there are no surrogates or substitutes. This clearly means that for a given case the perfect similimum can be only one. The outcome in a case shall entirely depend on how we have worked out the case to reach at the this perfect similimum.

By no means is this an easy task. It is indeed a very challenging and laborious task but at the same time quite interesting too. Once the case taking is done the most important symptoms observed in the case has to be logically rearranged according to their importance in the case to construct the totality of the case (discussed in detail later). This totality shall reflect an image which we call it as the image of sickness or portrait of the disease.

Once such an image is formed it has to be matched with the most similar image that a remedy shall reflect. That is image of sickness must perfectly fit in with the image of remedy. It must be kept in mind that there can be only one image possible for a person who is sick i.e., image of sickness can be only one for a given case however there can be such multiple conceptual images for a single remedy.

Sometimes we observe that the same remedy may fit in as the similimum for two persons having exactly opposite symptoms. This is because when the image of sickness is formed for these two cases there is a possibility that the same drug reflects both this images hence fitting in as the similimum. To summarize there are certain peculiarities in each patient which identifies him as an individual patient also there are some pecularities in each drug that identifies itself as an individual remedy. When these pecularities match the remedy thus fits in as the similimum for the given case.

"Every remedy has in itself a certain state of peculiarities that identifies it as an individual remedy, and the patient has also a certain state of peculiarities that identifies him as an individual patient, and so the remedy is fitted to the patient. No remedy must be given because it is in the list, for the list has only been made as a means of facilitating the study of that epidemic" (J T Kent)

Basis for selection of a remedy

The remedy must be selected always only based on the totality of the case. It must be kept in mind that presence of one symptom does not rule in favor of a remedy nor absence of one rule out a remedy. As we have discussed above the same remedy can have multiple conceptual images and it is beyond the capacity of the human brain to remember all such images reflected by a drug. When we study any drug from the materia medica an attempt has to be made to learn how to construct this image.

In acute cases the remedy is decided based on acute totality. There are several ways in which an acute totality can be constructed (discussed later in detail) depending upon what we have in the given case. However, in chronic cases a uniform approach has to be followed while constructing the totality which has been discussed in detail later in this book.

3. Suceptability, predisposition and Miasms (An introduction)

In Homeopathy susceptibility is considered as the general quality or capability of the living organism of receiving impressions; the power to react to stimuli.

Now let's try to understand this suceptability in detail.

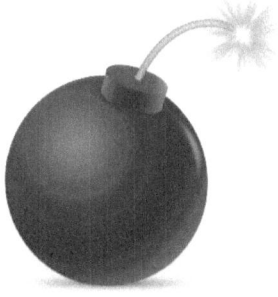

As you can see the above image is of a cracker bomb. This bomb shall not explode on its own but when it comes in contact with any source of fire then it shall explode causing damage and destruction.

When the same bomb is kept away or protected from any source of fire it shall continue to remain as it is, but it shall still have that tendency to cause an explosion when it comes in contact with any source of fire. This tendency makes it susceptible to cause an explosion and this susceptibility shall remain and cannot be removed.

This cracker bomb can be compared to the susceptibility that every individual has in him from within. Just like that destructive power of the cracker bomb comes into play only when its triggered by any source of fire, similarly the susceptibility within every individual comes into play only when it is triggred by any exciting factor. These exciting factors can come from various sources and a person can almost get exposed to these factors at any given point of time. However, when the person is healthy and his vitality is in order, the strong dynamic protective covering shall ensure that these triggering factors do not excite the susceptibility. It is the presence of this susceptibility that makes a person sick when the vitality is deranged resulting in causing physical symptoms.

So, when the dynamic protective covering becomes weak the negative dynamic influence acts upon the vital force and tends to cause its derangement. This derangement creates an imbalance which flows from the centre to the periphery and settles on the materlsitic plane at one or more parts which then makes those parts susceptible to cause disease realted to that particular part(s).

Often, we clinically observe that in many patients there is a family history of similar sufferings.

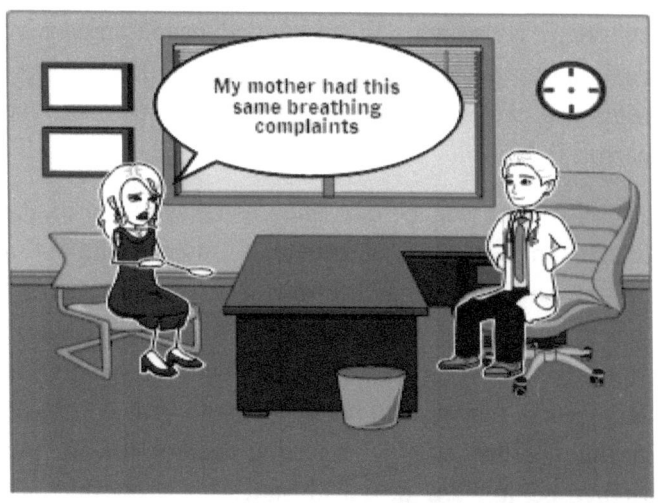

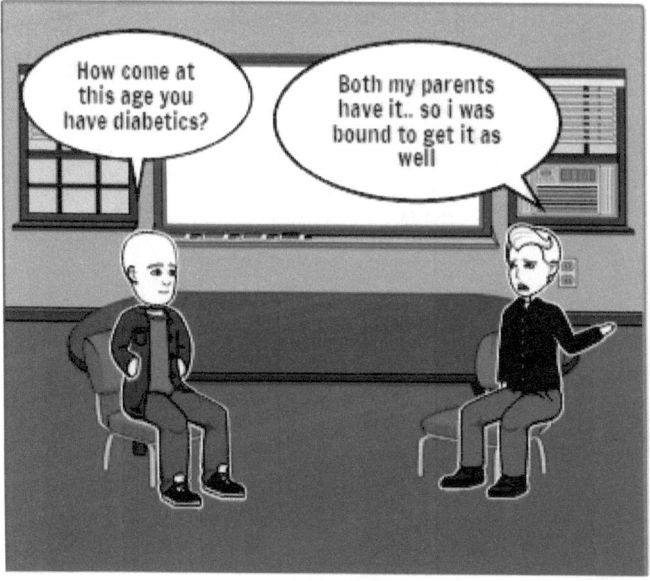

This susceptibility remains in a dormant state as long as the vitality is in order and the dynamic protective covering is strong. When the dynamic protective covering becomes weak and the vitality is deranged, the triggering factors excite the sucseptibiity to make the person sick.

So, disease can be explained as an outcome of the interaction between the individual susceptibility of a person and the triggering factors. These triggering factors can come into play only when the dynamic protective covering is weakened, and the vitality is deranged. A person shall not develop physical symptoms in the absence of this trigerring factors despite the vitality being in a deranged state. Let's consider an example to understand this statement:

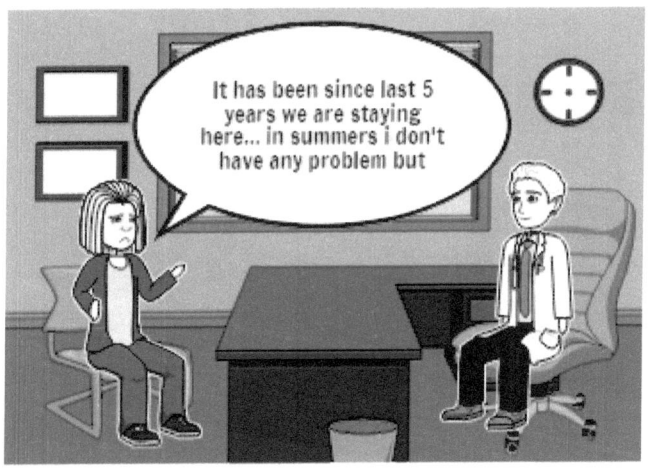

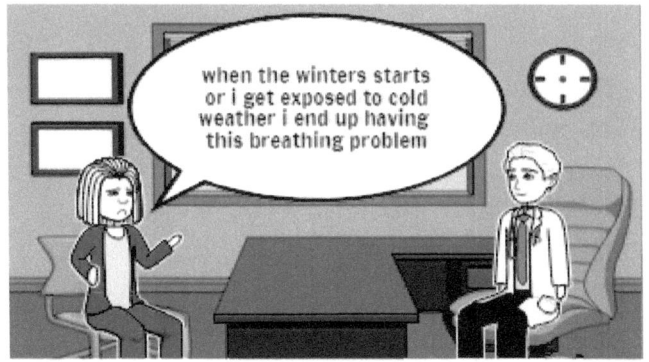

You must have observed some partients having asthmatic complaints for years together, but they have this problem only in winters or when they get exposed to cold weather. They remain absolutely fine in hot weathers and during summer season. Now in such cases it's not that their vitality is back to order during the summer season and it again gets deranged in winters but it's just the fact that patients having such chronic complaints remain free from the sufferings when they are not exposed to the exciting factors (in the above case cold). So, it's very clear that even though the vitality is in a deranged state and the patient is susceptible to develop physical symptoms still they remain free from these physical symptoms until they do not get exposed to the exciting factors which triggers the suscesptibility.

Weakened dynamic protective covering + deranged vital force = Increased susceptibility

Increased Susceptibility + Exposure to exciting factors = Physical symptoms

This individual susceptibility varies from person to person and also it varies in the same person under different situations. This clearly means that there are some factors upon which the susceptibility of a person depends upon. These factors include:

1) <u>Age:</u> The newborn infants and children have generally a high susceptibility but as their immunity builds with age their susceptibility tends to diminish (not unconditionally). Again, as the person grows old with this process of ageing the susceptibility also tends to increase. Hence, we see generally that small children and people in old ages are more prone to develop diseases as they have high susceptibility. Those children who are brought up dependent on allopathic medicines generally remain highly susceptibile even in their young age as because of such medications the general immunity fails to develop.

2) <u>Mental health:</u> Poor mental health which includes fear, sadness, depression, disappointments etc has a direct impact in lowering the strength of the dynamic protective covering therby people with such negative mental health tend to have high susceptibility. On the other hand, people who are mentally strong and positive generally have a very strong dynamic protection thereby lowering their susceptibility. We often hear people saying a healthy mind means a healthy body. Hence all sources which yield dynamic positive energies helps to keep the person healthy by adding to the

strength of dynamic protective covering therby lowring their susceptibility.

3) <u>Physical Hygeine:</u> Good physical hygiene and health helps to lower the susceptibility. On the other hand, malnutrition, starving etc tends to make the person sick by increasing the persons susceptibility. Unhealhy habits like cigerrate smoking, alcohol consumption etc also adds to the factors that increases this individual susceptibility.

4) <u>External environmental conditions</u>: Favourable external environmental conditions helps to keep a person health and fit thereby lowering his individual susceptibility whereas unfavourable external environmental conditions create a negative vibe which then lowers the strength of dynamic protective covering thereby making the person highly susceptible.

5) <u>Unusual physical or metal exhaustion:</u> Unusual heavy physical exertion or mental exhaustion tends to lower the strength of the dynamic protective covering thereby increasing the individual susceptibility.

So, as a general rule we can say that individual susceptibility is inversely proportional to the strength of the dynamic protective covering. The stronger the dynamic protective covering the weaker is the susceptibility and the weaker the susceptibility the weaker the chances of developing disease.

However, it also must be kept in mind that the above discussed factors affecting the susceptibility do not operate individually but all these factors affect in tandem and the outcome depends on the overall output of all the factors taken together.

Now the question is from where and when does this susceptibility come in an individual?

Every individual ever since birth is predisposed towards developing certain diseases. This predisposition is acquired from the parents and exits wthin an individual ever since his birth. It is this predisposition that makes a person susceptible.

This predisposition is acquired from the parents through something that we call it as the "Miasms". So bacically it is the miasms that is responsible for the predisposition and this predisposition inturn makes a person susceptible. Such a susceptible person when gets exposed to exciting factors tends to develop disease provided the vital force is in a deranged state.

When the vital force is in order despite having a predisposition and high susceptibility the person shall not fall sick even after getting exposed to exciting factors because the vital force in order ensures that the dynamic protective covering is strong enough not to allow the exciting factors to triger the susceptibility of an individual.

It also has to be kept in mind that the susceptibility cannot be removed, but can only be modified. This modification ensures that despite having exposed to exciting factors the person shall not develop disease. The suscpetibility depends directly on the strength of the dynamic protective covering. In children and in old peoples the strength of the dynamic protective covering remains weak hence such people are prone to develop diseases very often.

Any factor that contributes towards bringing down the strength of the dynamic protective covering increases the susceptibilty. On the other hand, those factors which retains or adds to the strength of the dynamic protective covering brings down the individual susceptibility.

Let's consider an example to understand this in a better way.

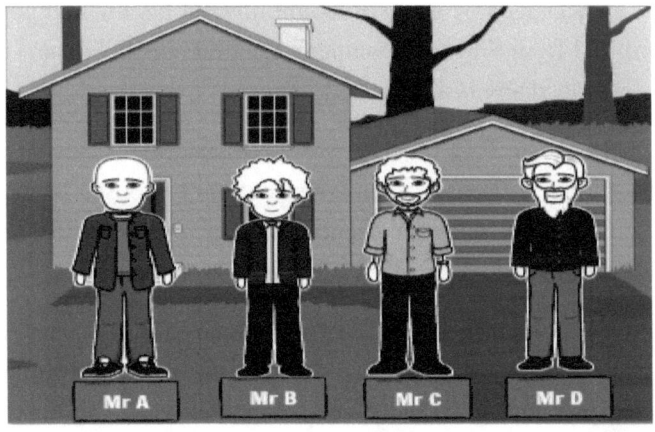

In the image above we have four people Mr A aged 35, Mr B aged 27, Mr C aged 57 and Mr D aged 64. Let's assume that all these four people are working in a factory where they get exposed to smell of harmful chemicals.

Mr A aged 35 has been working there since last 8 years and for past 7 years he did not had any probelm but since last 1 year he is suffering from respiratory disorder.

Mr B aged 27 has been working only since last 1 year and he is also suffering from respiratory disorder for last 5 months.

Mr C aged 57 has been working in the same company for last 30 years and is about to retire in next 1 year. He did not have any health problems for last 29 years but since last 1 year he developed migraine.

Mr D aged 64 has worked throughout his life and got retired from the same company six years back. He never developed any health realted issues.

If these four people are predisposed to develop respiratory diseases, then when they get exposed to the smell of the harmful chemicals, they are expected to develop the disease.

Mr A having worked in the company for 7 years did not develop the disease despite being susceptible because during all these years the vitality was in order and the dynamic protective covering was strong enough to prevent the exciting factors from trigerring his individual susceptiblity. Once these dynamic protective covering became weak and vital force got deranged the exposure to exciting factors trigerred the susceptibility to make the person sick.

Mr B developed the disease within first few months because he had the predisposition and that made him susceptible and since the dynamic protective covering was weak and vital force was in a deranged state immediate exposure to exciting factors trigerred the susceptibility to cause the disease.

Mr C has been working in the same company for almost 23 years and he remained quite healthy for all these years but towards the end he developed migraine and not respiratory disease. This is because he had no predisposition to develop respiratory diease and hence he was not susceptibe. His predispostion resulted in having a migraine as he was susceptible to develop the same.

Mr D had no predispotion for any of the diseases for which these harful chemicals would have acted as an exciting factor hence he never developed any health realted issues.

To summarize this introduction on susceptibilty, predisposition and miasms we can say that it is the maisms that is responsible for the predispostion and this predisposition makes a person susceptible and when such a susceptible person gets exposed to exciting factors, he falls sick.

Step by step approach to practice classical homoeopathy

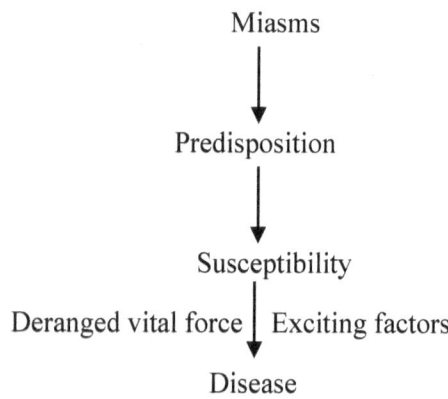

4. Case taking

Case taking is the art of collecting information about the patient. If practicing Homoeopathy can be compared to a journey, then the starting point from where the journey begins is the "case taking" and our destination is the end point being the "cure".

It's said that "case taking is an art and a well taken case is as good as half cured." This sentence emphasizes the need to master this art of case taking if we wish to get the expected result in each and every case. When we compare the process of case taking to an art it must be kept in mind that an art is something that cannot be learned or taught unless one dosen't have the interest to learn and master it. Here in this chapter we shall go through the various aspects of case taking in detail.

To begin with we have to first understand that case taking is not just about collecting the symptoms from a patient. It is all about understanding the patient as a whole. So, let's first try to understand the aims and objectives of a detailed case taking:

Aims and objectives: In acute cases

Acute cases are those which have a sudden onset, a rapid progress and a definite course. They tend end in either death or recoevery once it has runout its course.

From this definition it's very clear that while handling acute cases the remedy has to be decided quickly in the shortest possible time. Here we shall consider only those self limiting acute cases which are not fatal. The fatal diseases are discussed elsewhere in this book.

The aim and objectives of case taking in a self limiting, non fatal acute case are as follows:

a) To identify the exciting cause or root cause for onset of the present acute complaints

b) To look for the characteristic symptoms belonging to the patient in the given case.

c) To isolate any alterations in the mental plane or in physical generalities that is not common to the disease.

d) To list down all the acute deviations from health along with its intensity.

e) To arrive at a clinical diagnosis based on the symptoms observed.

f) To identify the presence of any maintaining cause for the given case.

Managing acute cases

As we have just discussed acute cases are usually self limiting. They have a sudden onset, rapid progress and a definite course. They tend to terminate either in recovery or death once it has runout its course. In this section we shall discuss as to how to manage an acute case that is non fatal. Have a look at the graph shown below which shows the progress of an acute case. The vertical line indicates the intensity of symptoms whereas the horizontal line indicates the number of days.

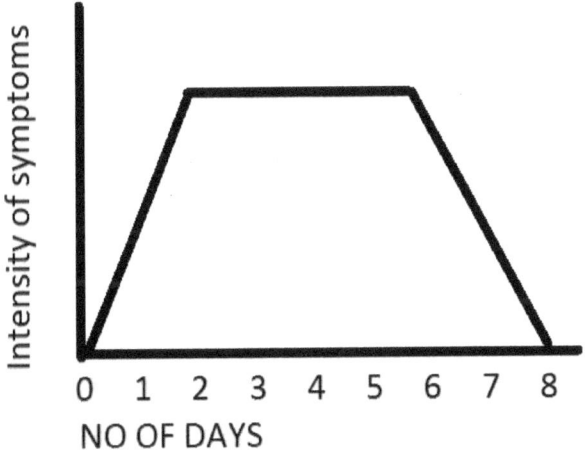

As you can observe in the above graph that the acute diseases has a sudden onset and within few hours the intensity of symptoms increases to reach a peak level where it remains as it is for a few days and then gradually the intensity reduces as the disease runsout its course finally recovering completely.

This clearly means that in such acute cases even if no medicine is given the patient shall completely recover after the disease runs out its course.

There are basically two ways to manage such acute cases. One way is to by any means bring down the intensity of the present complaints so that while under medication the patient will feel a little better and once the disease has run out its course the patient is bound to recover completely. The beow graph explains the same.

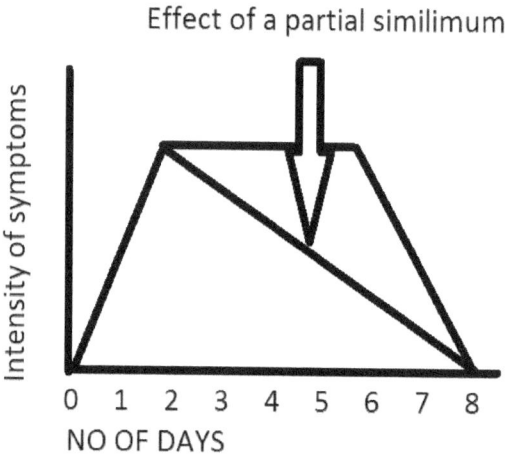

Effect of a partial similimum

In the above graph we can see the effect when a remedy is given to bring down the intensity of symptoms. As you can observe under the influence of such a remedy the patient can be made to feel a little better but still the disease shall run out its course and it will take around one week for the patient to recover completely.

This kind of results can be seen clinically when a remedy is prescribed based on the common symptoms, when multiple remedies are given or when tinctures and commercial combination products are prescribed.

With such prescriptions one may be able to bring down the intensity of symptoms a little down but still the disease would run out its course.

The other option to manage an acute case is to abort the progress of it. Have a look at the graph below:

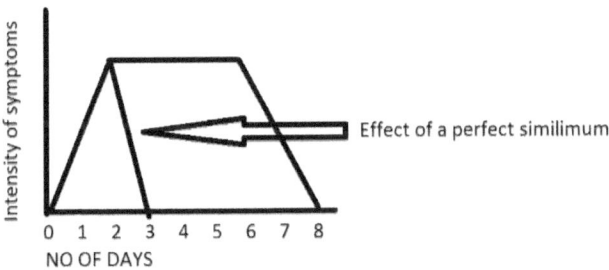

The above graph shows the effect of a perfect similimum. As we can see the perfect similimum will not allow the disease to run out its course and its progress is aborted helping the patient to recover in double quick time. The abilty to abort the progress of such acute cases is something that only our remedies can do and if we all make an attempt to learn as to how to achieve this kind of results that shall definitely give our system an upper hand over the conventional system of medicine.

Here is the reference for what has been explained above.

"Hahnemann says that all acute diseases should be aborted.

Why should we not expect to do this if Hahnemann did so a hundred years ago?

Why call ourselves Homoeopathicians if we cannot do as well as Hahnemann did?

Why not offer this as the test of our ability and skill, and consciously admit that we must abort all acute diseases or cease to call ourselves homoeopathicians?

There can be no better test for our work and for our position than to announce to the world that we do this, if we do it and let all others compare their work and stand or fall by the test of clinical experience," (Lesser writings by J T Kent)

"Homoeopathicians abort all acute diseases-what do others accomplish?

It only remains for us to educate the people so they will know what to expect, and what can be done, and who can do it.

But first the education must begin with the physician, so that he can meet the requirements.

Some will say "We do not believe it," which simply means that they have not seen such results, and this only signifies that they do not know how to apply the remedies homeopathically.

Then let the education begin at home. That there are many professed Hahnemannians who are not doing this work in this way is no reason for our silence.

It is enough to know that Hahnemann did it, that many others are doing it, that we should all do it. If we cannot do so, let us give up our pretensions." (Lesser writings J T Kent)"

To abort the progress of an acute disease the prescription has to be based on the totality of symptoms and this totality has to be constructed based on quality symptoms of the patient and not on the basis of the disease symptoms.

Collecting the information in an acute case

Collecting the required information or case taking in an acute is always a challenging task for every homeopath. In such acute cases mostly, the patient expects to get a quick relief and wants to have the medicines without much questioning being done. So, if we wish to abort the progress of any acute disease, we need to focus on collecting only the quality symptoms in the shortest possible time.

When we talk about the quality symptoms especially in such acute cases, we are referring only to the symptoms of the patient that shall guide us to construct the totality. The following symptoms deserves to get more importance if noticed and well marked provided they are very striking, strange or peculiar to the given case conditions.

1) <u>Look for any altered disposition at mental level</u>: We have to keep in mind that patients are not aware about what we need from them to make a successful prescription so mostly they will not tell the information that we require but instead they tend to narrate only those common set of symptoms as they are used to narrating infront of an allopathic doctor. They usually give priority to only the physical symptoms which came at the end and will omit, although unintentionally the symptoms observed in the beginning. Let's show you an example:

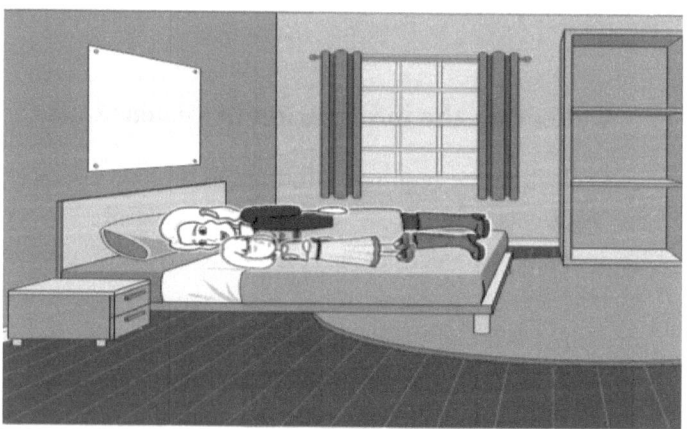

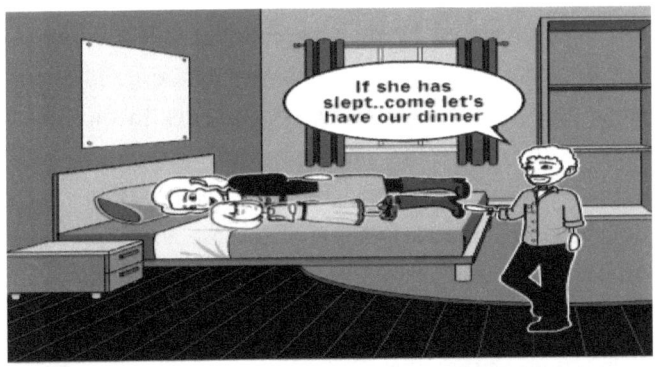

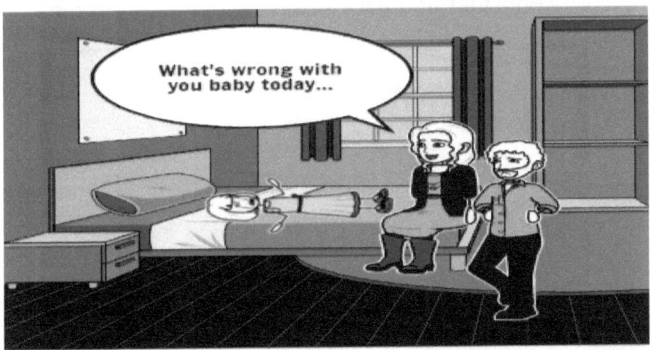

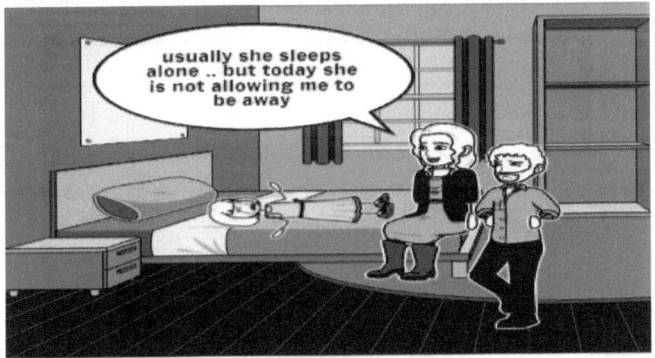

In this example it's very clearly getting reflected that there is some devaiation from the normal behavior for that child. She does not want to be alone. This deviation has been observed by their parents but still they would not think about consulting a doctor as the child at this stage do not have any physical complaints. In such cases they prefer to wait, until physical symptoms shall appear. Basically, they fail to realize that these deviations are the early signs of disease and if managed properly at this stage the physical symptoms won't appear at all. In other words, the diease can be aborted.

Let's consider another example:

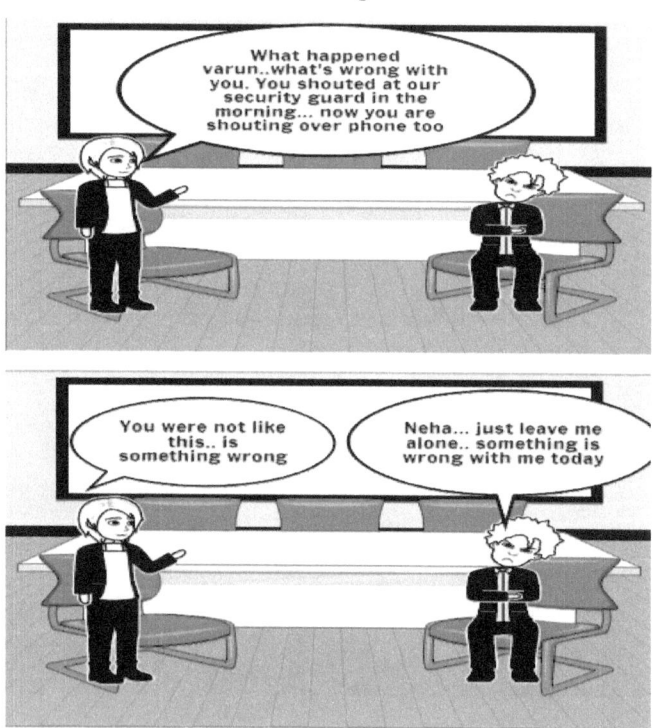

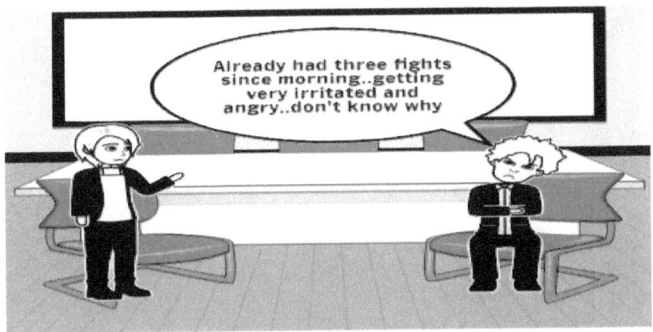

As you can clearly observe in the above example too lot of deviations are noticed at the mental plane which indicates the flow of imbalance, but physical symptoms are yet to appear. These symptoms which indicate the early signs of derangement are very important for us in forming the totality.

2) <u>Hunt for the causative factor because of which the acute complaints have been triggered:</u> In managing acute cases the triggering factor or the causative factor has atmost importance. If they are found and are striking, they deserve to get most value. Usually in acute cases such a trigerring factor can easily be traced as in many cases the patient's themselves shall disclose it even without asking for it. Here is an example

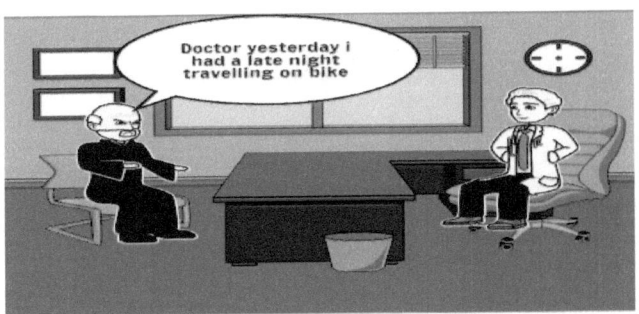

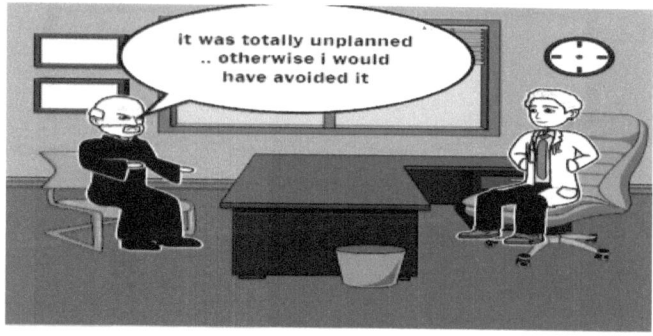

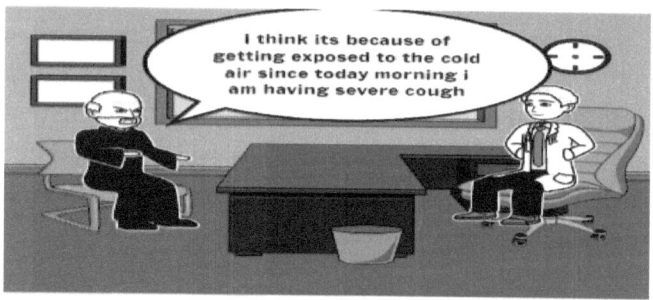

In the above example as we can see the triggering factor was getting exposed to cold which is clearly been mentioned by the patient. In such cases these causative triggering factors deserves to get considered on priority while constructing the totality. In some cases, the patient may not be aware of the triggering factor, but skillful questioning can help us to find such triggering factors. Here is an example

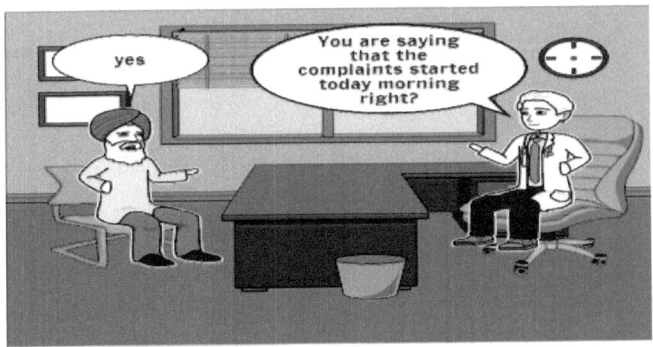
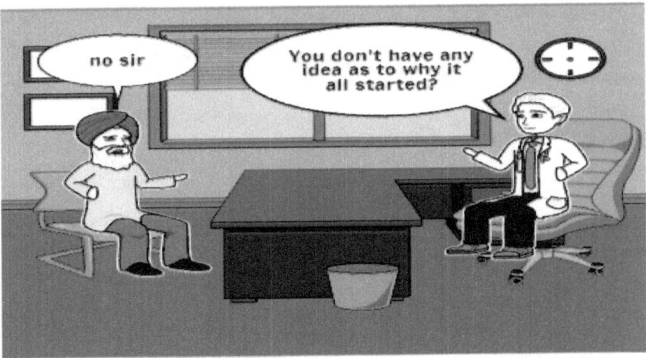
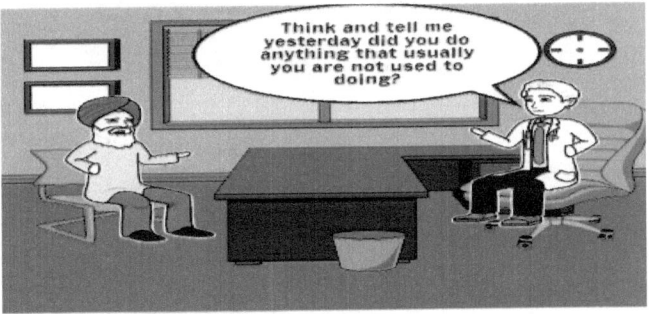

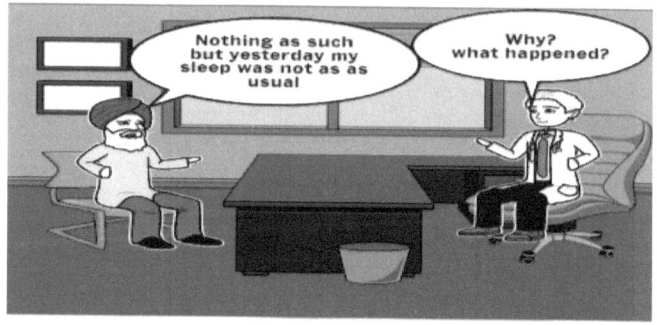

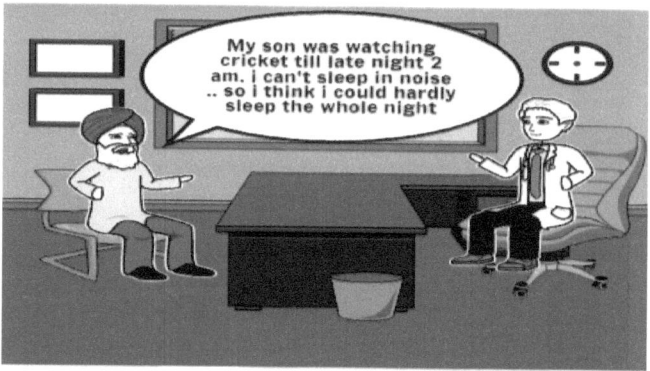

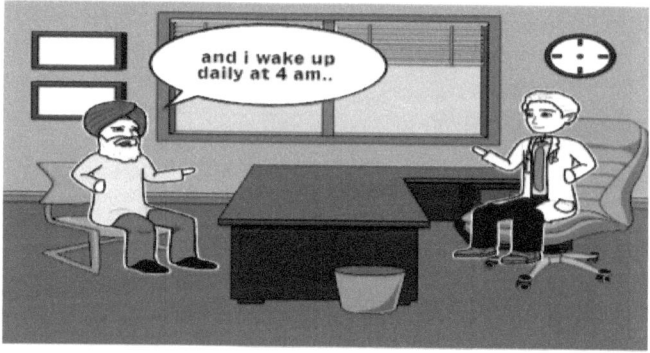

A skillful questioning is very essential to reach at the exciting or root cause for the onset of such acute complaints. Mostly the cause in such cases would be something that the patient had to encounter before few hours from the onset of complaints. A through enquiry into all the past activities done a few hours before would help us to get a clarity on the real exciting or root cause.

3) <u>Altered physical generals which are not common to the condition or disease</u>: Physical generals include symptoms related to appetite, desires, aversions, thirst, sleep, symptoms related to all natural discharges including perspiration and menstruation, bowel habits and urination. If any alteration is found related to these physical generals which is strange and not common to the present condition or disease, then those symptoms are of high importance. Here is an example:

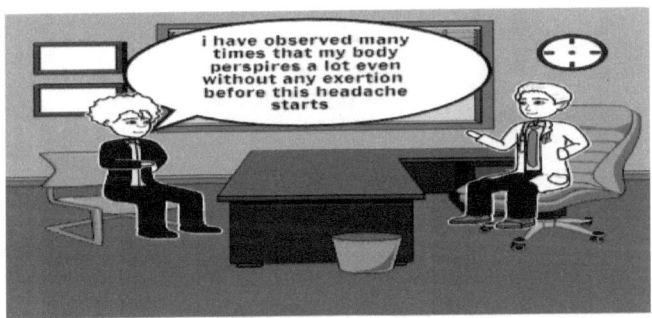

Increased perspiration before the onset of complaints is a very important physical general that is strange and peculiar to the individual hence such groups of symptoms have high value. At the same time a person who has had profuse diarrhea and severe vomiting when brought for consultation is in a severily dehydrated state. In such a state we expect that the person will have excessive thirst. Incresed thist in such cases although is a altered physical general but in this scenario it is something that is expected to be present. Hence it then loses its value. However, in such cases if we find that the person is still thirstless then that becomes peculiar and strange giving it high value.

4) <u>Characteristic particulars</u>: All those particular symptoms that are uncommon, strange and peculiar have great importance in forming the acute totality. So, while taking an acute case one need to hunt for these characteristic particulars which may be present in the form of specific modality or in the form of any concomitant. Here is an example:

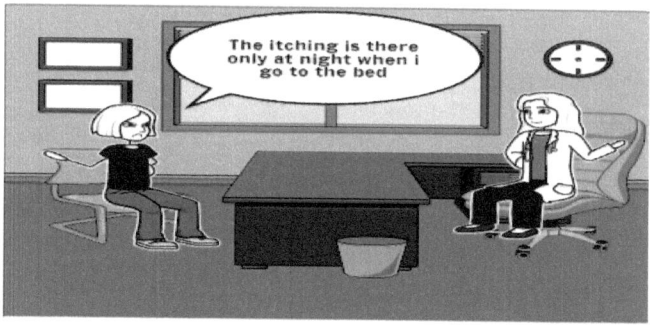

5) <u>Common symptoms:</u> Ideally it is not advisible to base a prescription based only on the common symptoms of the disease. However, in some acute cases only the symptoms common to the disease may be prominent. In such cases prescription can be made taking into account the group of symptoms having highest intensity. It also has to be kept in mind that such a prescription shall only help to bring down the intensity of symptoms.

Acute totality:

In an acute case the totality can be constructed in a number of ways. It will depend on what kind of quality symptoms we have in the given case. As a general rule the below mentioned hierarchy can be kept in mind while constructing an acute totality

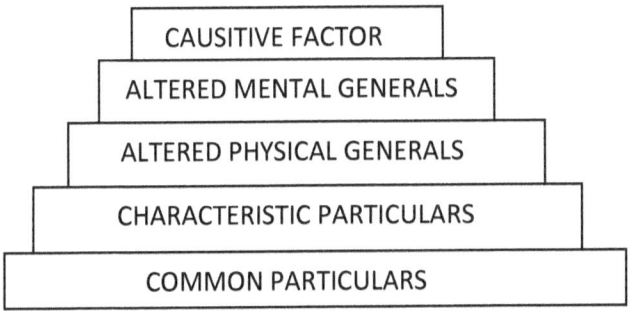

Just like an artist mixes his colors and selects the ideal combination as per the need or just like an architect designs his creativity similarly a physician should also use his own logic in an artistic way to construct the totality.

So, depending on what is present in a given case to construct the totality, accordingly the totality may differ.

Art and skill of taking an acute case

The output of case taking and what information we have at the end of case taking shall depend on the individual skill and art of taking it. This shall vary from physician to physician depending on their skill and art of questioning and observing. Here are some basic guidelines that a physician should keep in mind while taking an acute case.

1) In acute cases usually patients are quite desperate to get the medicines in the shortest possible time. Prolonged case taking in such situations can make the patient iriirated and angry. Care should be given to ensure the "comfort level" of the patient.

2) Usually in acute cases the changes that occur are quite recent and prominent. In most of the cases the patient shall readily give us the information about the most dominant symptoms which is causing the most discomfort to the patient. We have to carefully listen to the statement made by the patient because apart from collecting the symptoms that are prominent the way a person makes the statement, their facial expression many a times suggests their mentality, reaction or response towards the recently developed physical symptoms. Such reactions are related to that individual alone hence becomes very important for us. Let's consider an example:

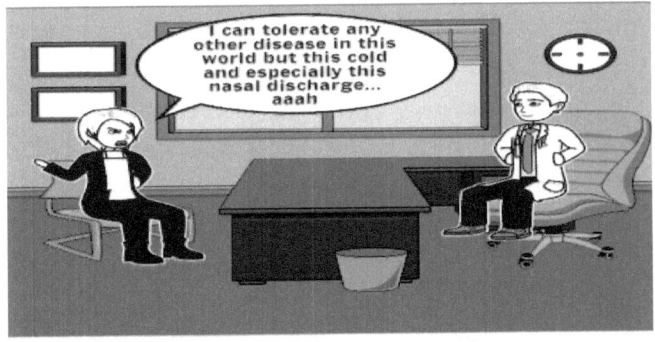

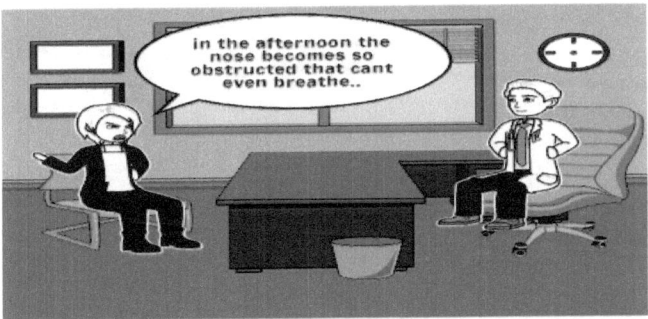

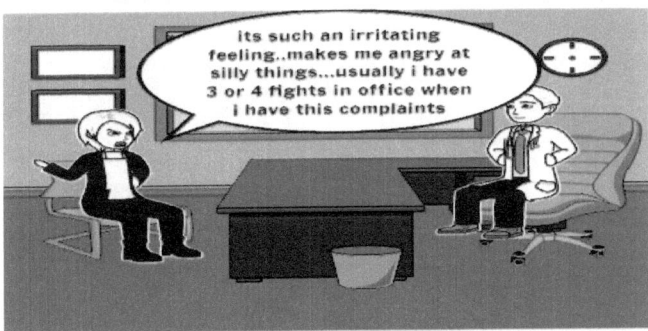

Now as you can observe from the above conversation, we have got few important physical symptoms and its modalities but at the same time along with that we got an altered symptom at mental level which indicates the response of that particular individual towards his disease. The symptoms coming out of such individual reactions have great importance in forming the totality. Let's consider yet another example of a person having the same complaints as above but totally a different reaction at mental level:

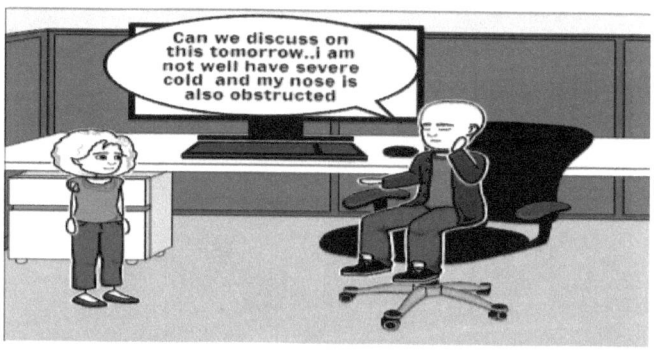

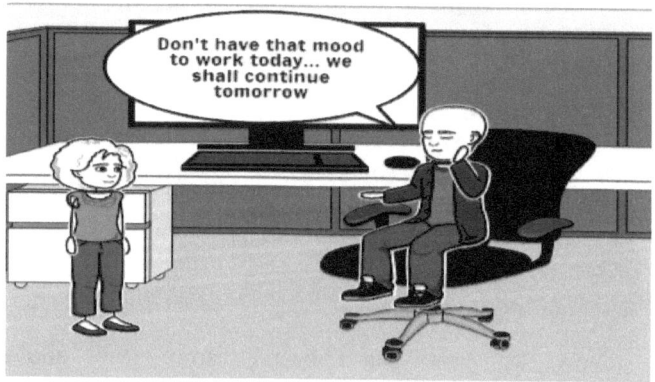

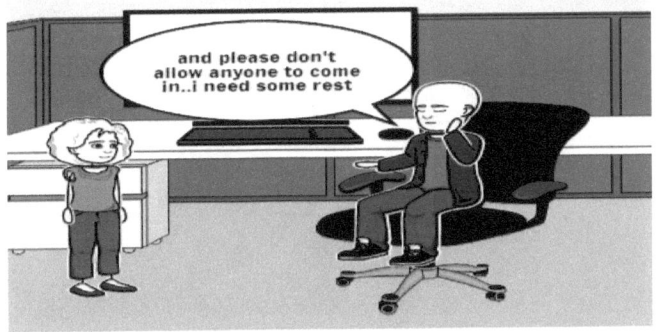

As it can be seen in both these examples the physical complaints are similar but the person reaction to it is totally different at mental level. These individualistic reactions needs to be traced while forming the totality.

Sometimes the patients themselves reflect this mentality by the way they way they narrate their complaints but in some cases to traceout this we need to frame our questions in an intelligent way as shown below:

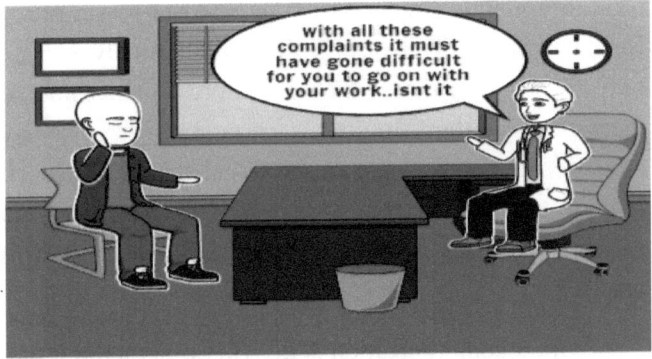

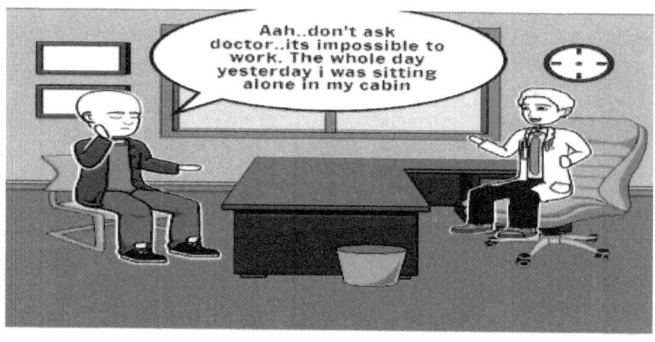

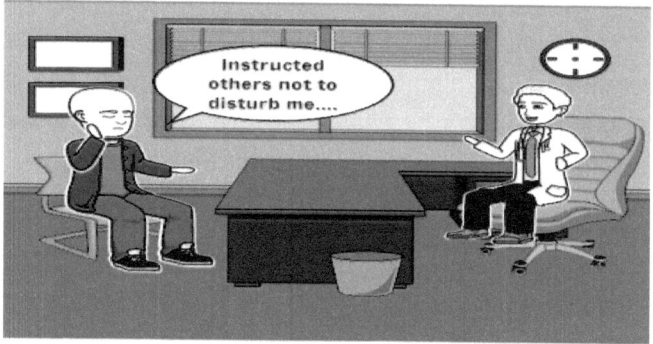

It must be kept in mind that the patients do not know what information we need from to base our prescription. Hence in most of the cases they shall usually narrate only those symptoms which are more troublesome to them or which they are used to narrating in front of any other doctor. So, we have an additional challenge in such cases to tactfully traceout what exactly we need from the patient. This tact and art can be mastered only with practice.

3) Good communication skill: This is something that each and every homeopath has to develop in them while preparing themselves for a case taking. It has to be kept in mind that people usually consulting a doctor come

with a negative mentality or negative frame of mind. In such situations if we learn to impart little positivity to the patient by the way we interact with them, shall play a vital role in speedy recovery.

4) Keen observation: It's said that in Homeopathy we treat the patient and not his disease. This means that it's the peculairties of the patient that guide us towards the right similimum. A physician needs to have a keen observation skill to trace out these peculiarities. The peculiarities may be expressed in various ways. It may be expressed in the movements that patient makes or may be expressed on his face. Sometimes even by-standers reveal these peculiarities while the case taking is been done. Here is an example:

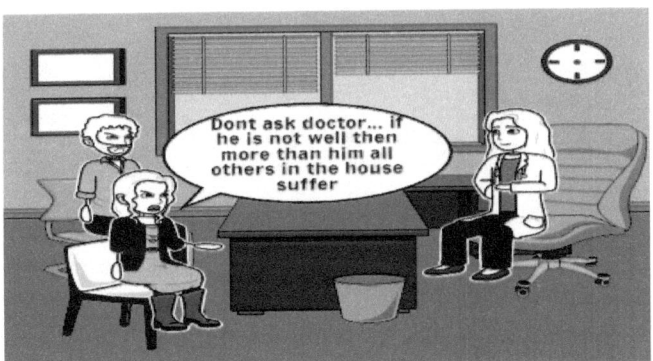

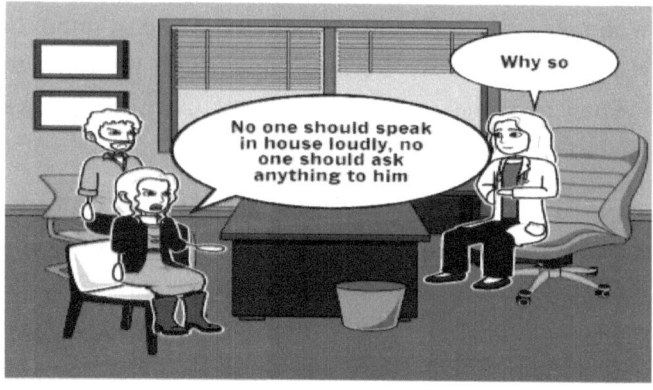

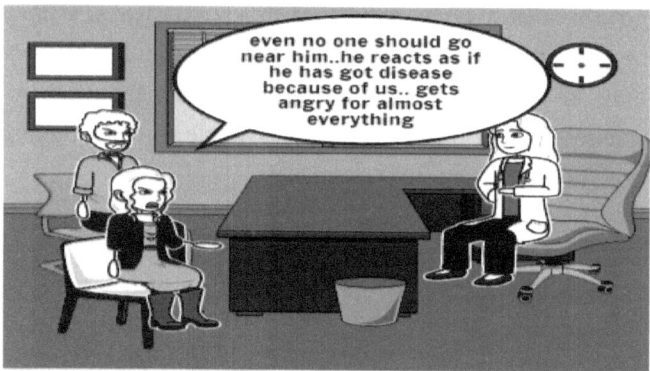

As shown in the above example the individual pecularities and reactions has to be traced in each and every given case to construct the perfect totality. It has to be kept in mind that the totality is for the patient as a whole and not limited to the disease ultimate or the part of body or organ affected.

Guidelines and instructions for take a case

Hahnemann has given very clear guidelines and instructions for taking a case in the aphorisms 83-104. Let's discuss on these instructions and guidelines in detail:

Aphorism 83

"This individualizing examination of a case of disease, for which I shall only give in this place general directions, of which the practitioner will bear in mind only what is applicable for each individual case, demands of the physician nothing but freedom from prejudice and sound senses, attention in observing and fidelity in tracing the picture of the disease"

It's very clear from the above aphorism that the instructions and guidelines given in these following aphorisms shall only give an overall idea as to how the individual case in hand has to be handled. It totally depends on the practitioner to decide keeping in mind these guidelines and instructions as to what is needed best for the given case and which approach should one adopt to trace out the required information about the patient. These instructions and guidelines are like the traffic rules that one learns from the driving school. Just like while driving a car these traffic rules has to be obeyed similarily while taking a case these guidelines and instructions has to be obeyed too depending upon the suitability and need of the case in hand.

This aphorism also describes the qualities that a physician needs to be equipped with in order to perform this task of taking a case in an artistic way. These qualities include

Freedom from Prejudice: Prejudice means to have a preconceived opinion about something that is not based on reason or actual experience. A Homoeopathic physician should always be free from any kind of prejudice and his actions, beliefs, observations and interpretations should be based strictly on proper reasoning and actual experience.

It is very important for each and every physician to relaise as to what can make him prejudiced and how fatal this can turn out to be for a physician. Prejudice comes when one has a preconceived opinion or predecided conclusion about something. As far as Homoepathic case taking is concerned the things that usually tend to make a physician prejudiced include:

1) <u>Having a list of remedies in mind for various clinical conditions</u>: It is now a days a common practice to memorize and remember in mind a set of remedies for a given clinical condition. People tend to list best remedies for asthma, arthritis, migraine etc. When one has this kind of list in their mind it shall make them prejudiced and then once the clinical diagnosis is made the physician only thinks about selecting a remedy from the list that he already has in his mind for that given clinical condition. Instead of observing carefully as to what is there in the case that belongs to the patients the

physician starts thinking about mounting a remedy from the list that he remembers upon the given case.

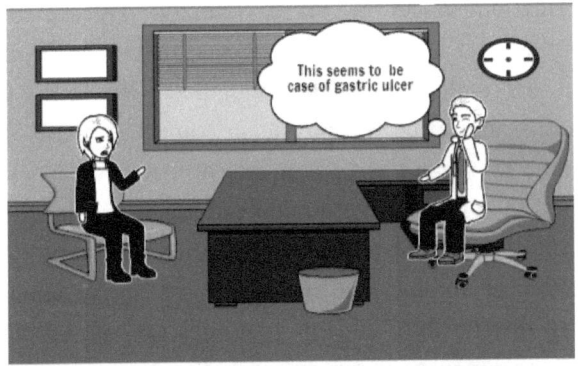

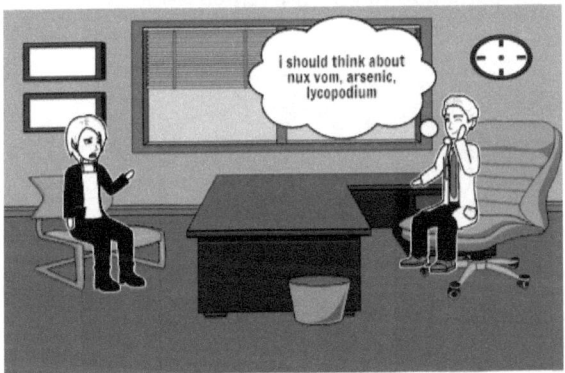

This prejudice leads him to think about the possibility of only those few set of remedies that he remembers for the given clinical condition and the chances are high that he shall miss out the prefect similimum and end up selecting a partial one.

2) <u>Memorized keynotes or fragments of remedy in mind</u>: As it has been already discussed that our materia medica contains such a vast informantion and knowledge that it becomes practically impossible for a human brain

to remember all those and usually many of us tend to remember only a few keynotes or few fragments of information about a given remedy. Having these keynotes and memorized fragments of remedy in mind shall also make a physician prejudiced. While the case taking is going on, if a physician come across any such keynote or memorized fragments of a remedy from the patient then he shall get prejudiced regarding the choice of remedy and his further questioning shall only be to confirm or mount that remedy upon the patient. By doing this he may end up forcing a set of symptoms upon the patient to justify the remedy select.

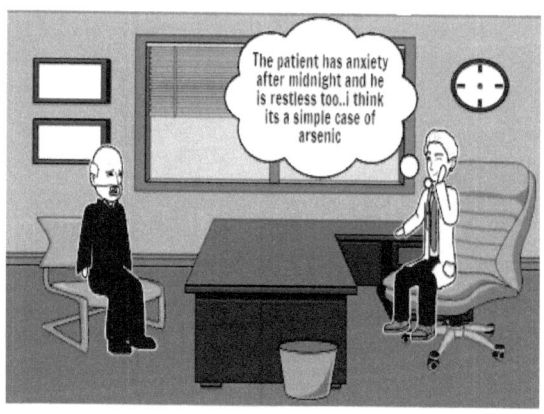

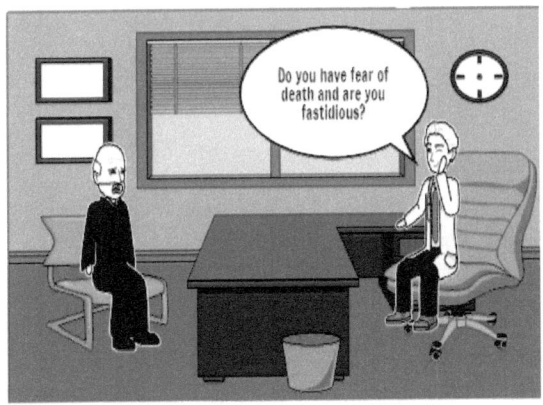

Such prejudice while framing the questions also shall lead to fatal error and the physician may end up selecting the wrong remedy.

3) <u>Lack of interpretation skill</u>: Interpretation means the action of explaining or understanding the meaning of something. Interpretation is also an art and a Homoeopathic physician should master this art of interpretation without which there are chances that he may become prejudiced. The statement made by the patient or something that a physician observes in the patient has to be cross checked to rule out all posibilities before reaching at a conclusion. If he admits blindly each and every statement made by the patient, they he may get misguided under prejudice. Let's consider an example:

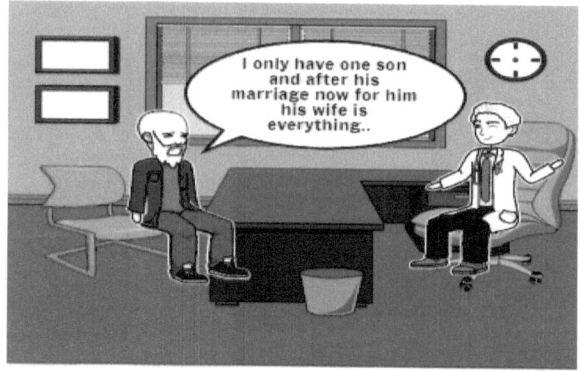

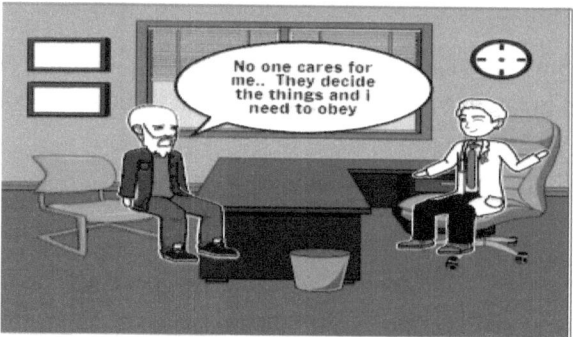

In the above case from the statement made by the patient it gives an impression that the patient is having "Forsaken" feeling but the same feeling was not geeting reflected either in his eyes nor in his facial exppression. Instead of getting prejudiced and jumping into considering "forsaken" rubric when his son was consulted the entire picture changed as follows:

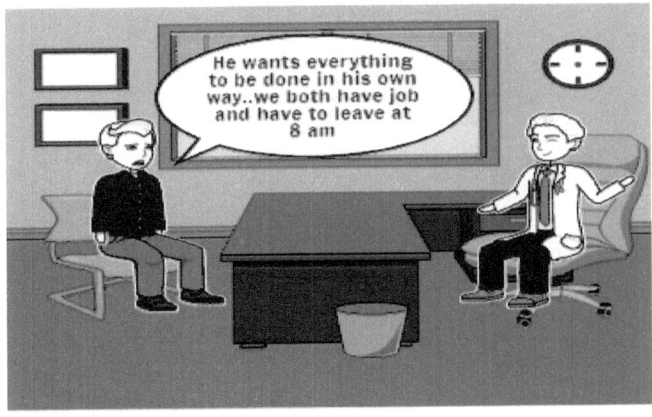
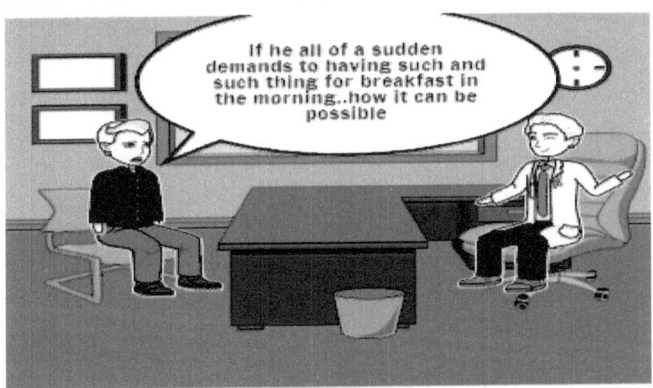

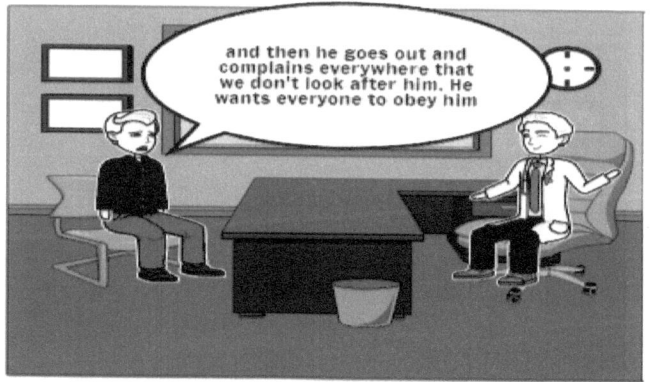

Sometyimes the statements made by the patients can be misleading and if admitted as it is out of prejudice then one may again end up in selecting the wrong remedy.

Sound senses: A physician should always have the sound senses to carefully observe and notice any change or pecularity however minor it may be. When he sees a patient, he has to pay careful attention to oserve his behaviour and facial expressions. Many times, the pecularities that belongs to the individual patient and his mental state often gets reflected in his actions or through his facial expression.

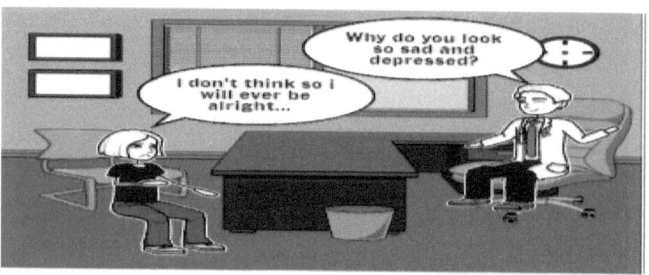

The physician may also be able to take a note of any smell while he takes the case or examines the patient. Such observations shall also help him to form the portrait of the sickness.

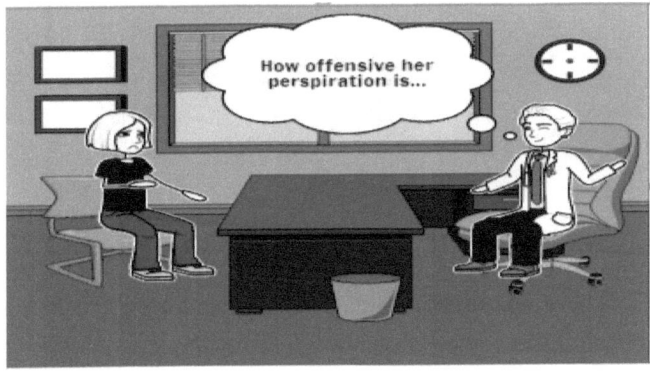

Attention in observing: A physician has to give careful attention to observe each and every minute fact about the patient. Such careful observations and its correct interpretations can be very useful for a physician in forming the totality. One such example is given below:

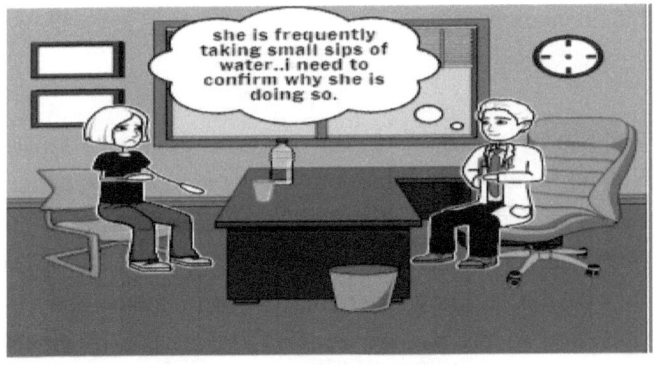

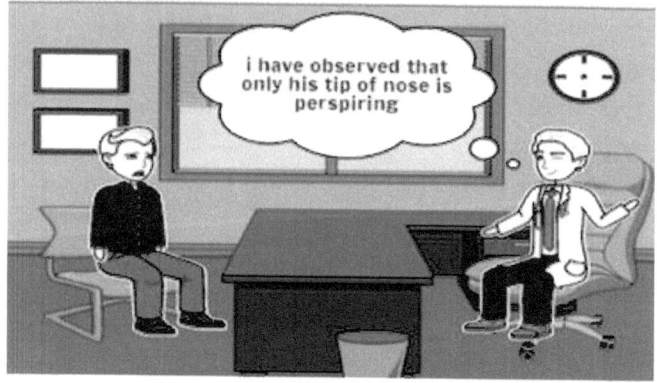

There are several facts that can be traced out if the physician has good observation skills like

Anxiety, panic, tension

Depression, disppointment and despair

Anger, irritation and frustration

Impatience, confusion and absent mindedness

A physician should also carefully observe the patients body language, the way he is communuicating and also his facial expressions.

Fidelity in tracing the picture of the disease: Fidelity means faithfulness to a person, cause, or belief, demonstrated by continuing loyalty and support. A physician should also be faithful to his patient and loyal to what he is doing extending his full support and co-operation to the patient while taking a case. He should not be in a hurry to run through the case but instead should devote as much time as possible to listen carefully and to understand his patient as a whole.

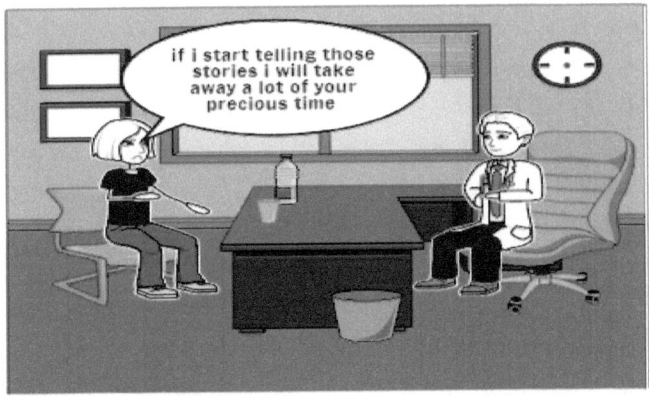

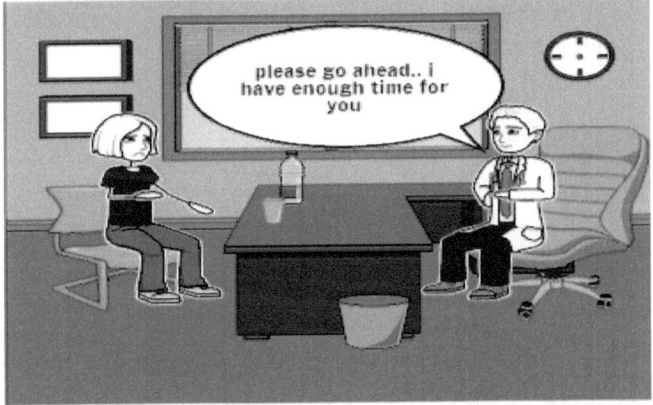

Such an assurance from the physician's side shall ensure that the patient develops a complete trust and faith upon the physician, and he shall then open up to describe his personal details as well.

Aphorism 84

"The patient details the history of his sufferings; those about him tell what they heard him complain of, how he has behaved and what they have noticed in him; the physician sees, hears, and remarks by his other senses what there is of an altered or unusual character about him. He writes down accurately all that the patient and his friends have told him in the very expressions used by them. Keeping silence himself he allows them to say all they have to say, and refrains from interrupting them1 unless they wander off to other matters. The physician advises them at the beginning of the examination to speak slowly, in order that he may take down in writing the important parts of what the speakers say."

1 Every interruption breaks the train of thought of the narrators, and all they would have said at first does not again occur to them in precisely the same manner after that.

This aphorism clearly instructs a physician to pay attention to what the patient is speaking and refrain himself from interupting the patient as long as he is speaking about himself or his complaints.The free flow of information from the patient's side can only be expected if a comfort level is given to him to speak openly and freely without any interruption. Unwanted interruption may break the flow of speech and the real expressions and emotions may not come out.

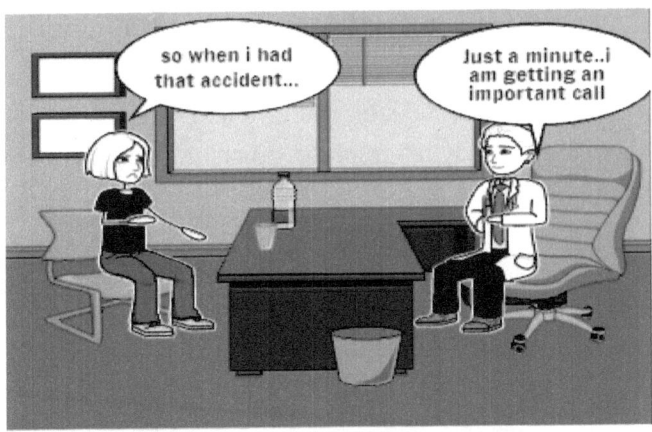
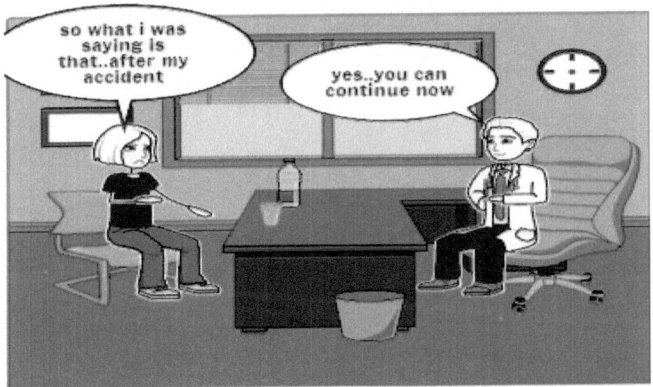
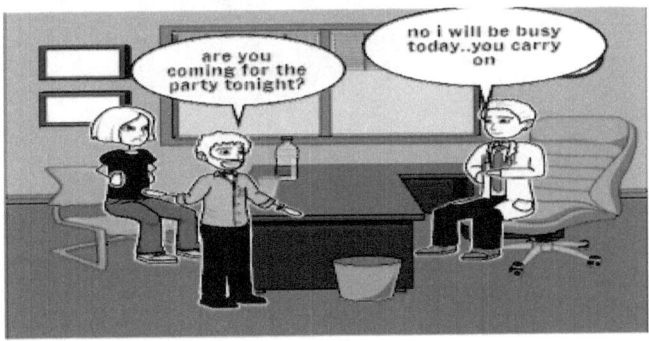

But again, if the patient starts talking about things that are not related to him, his surroundings or his complaints and something that is of no use to a physician then he can mildy interrupt the patient to bring him back to the topic of concern.

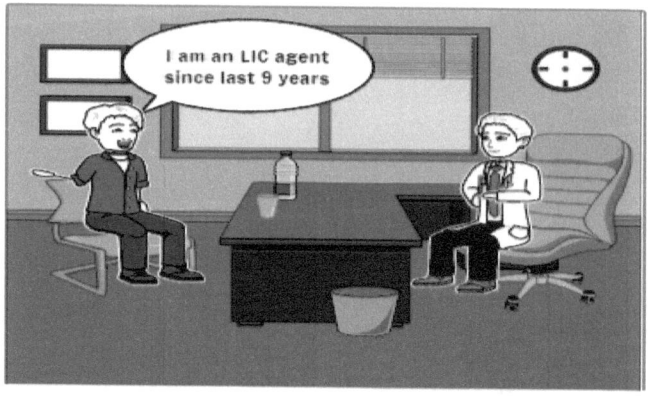

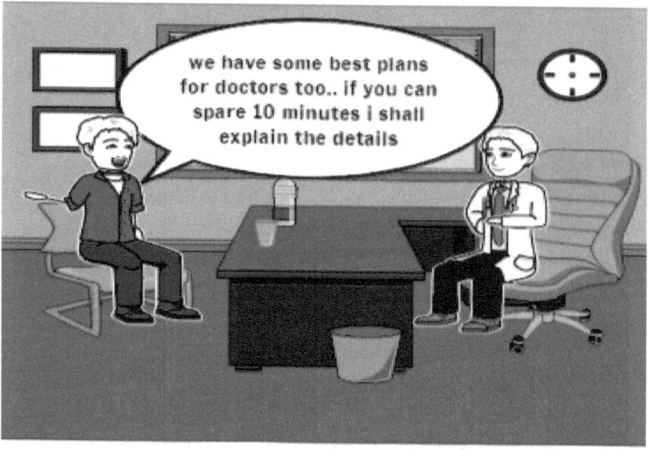

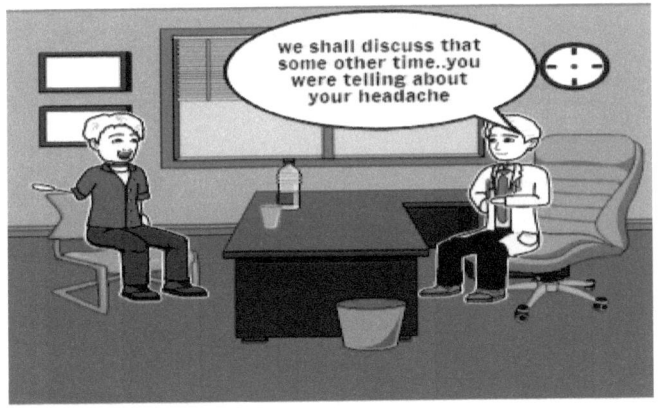

In many cases careful listening has got its own therapeutic value. We often read that case taking is an art and a well taken case is as good as half cured. In todays era everyone is in race. Race to make their future secure, race to earn something, race to survive etc. No one basically has time for others and in such a situation when we give our time and dedication to listen to the patient, his complaints, understand his emotions, feelings he gets so impressed that a positive vibe is transmitted to him that gives a feeling of relief and satisfaction to him making him feel 50% better. He then goes to disclose all those details which may be very useful for us in tracing the portrait of the sickness. This rapport and support build with the patient always helps to cure the patient in a much shorter time. Very often at the end of a detailed case taking patients often says this:

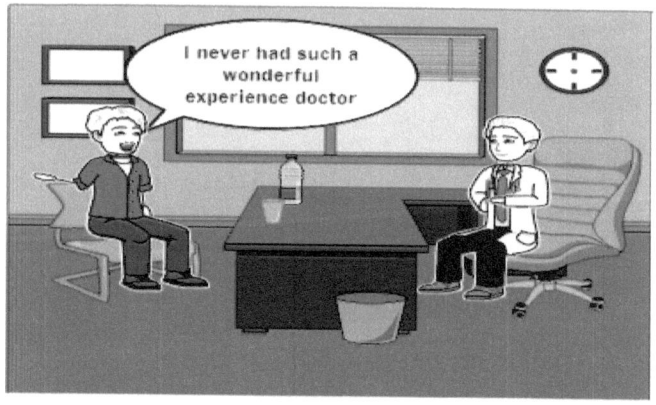
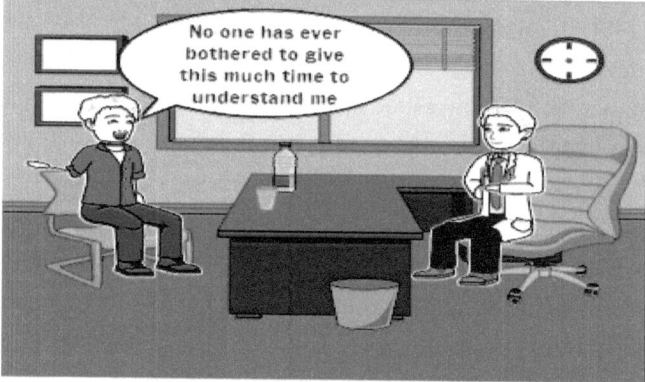
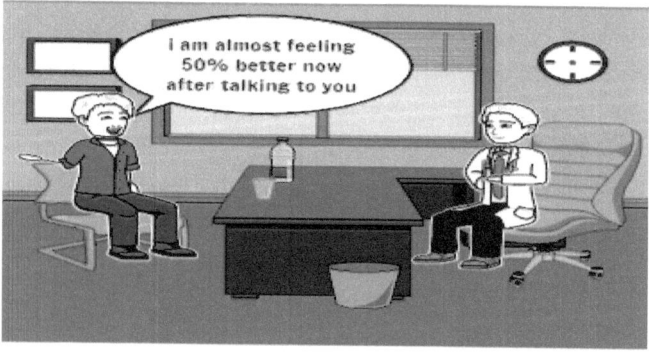

Ideally the physician while actively listening to the patient should acknowledge the feelings of the patients and show some interst and curiosity towards understanding not just the patient's sufferings but also the patient as a whole.

Sometimes a lot of important information is disclosed by the bystanders too. The bystander is a person who accompanies with the patient. If he is very close to the patient then he shall be in a position to narrate the changes especially at mental level that has been observed in the patient and also shall be able to guide the physician in understanding the normal disposition of the patient and his behaviour.

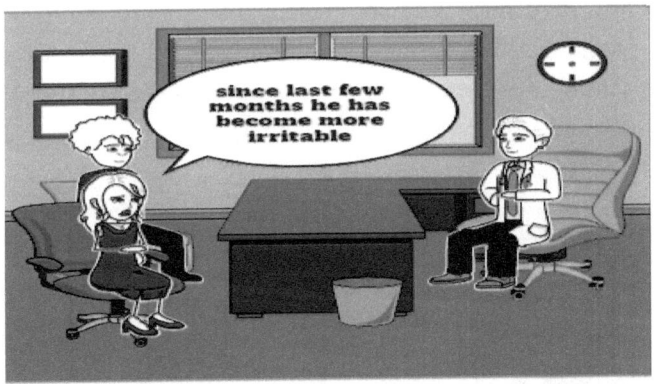

In short, a physician should collect the maximum information about his patient from all possible sources which includes what the patient is telling, what is been told by his bystanders and the individual observations of the physician himself.

Aphorism 85:

"He begins a fresh line with every new circumstance mentioned by the patient or his friends, so that the symptoms shall be all ranged separately one below the other.

He can thus add to any one, that may at first have been related in too vague a manner, but subsequently more explicitly explained."

Usually when a patient having multiple complaints starts narrating them, he does so in a very vague manner as he is not aware of what we need from him to make a sucessful prescription. In such a case the patient is allowed to speak without interruption all the complaints that he may be having. The physician has to note down each of these complaints one below the other. He should start a fresh line for every new complaint narrated by the patient.

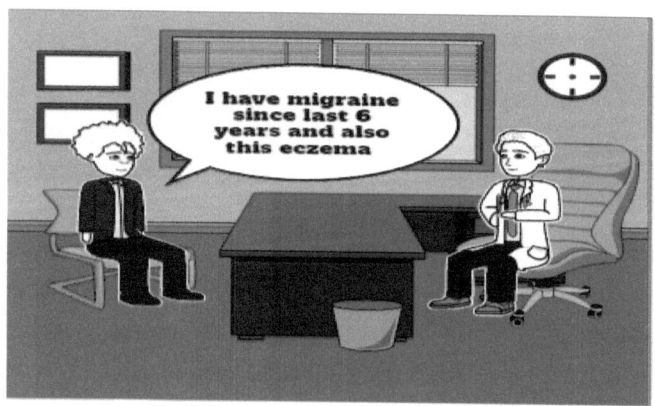

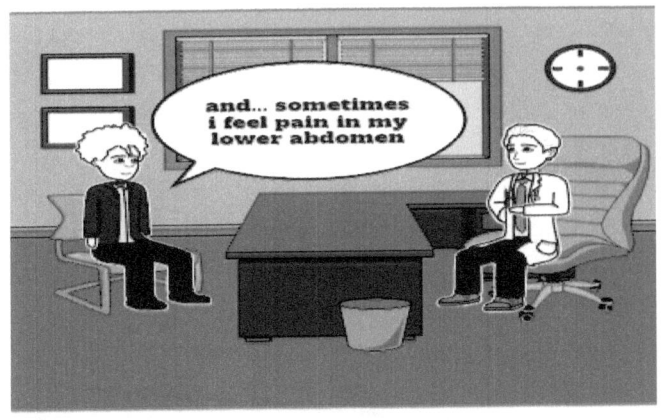

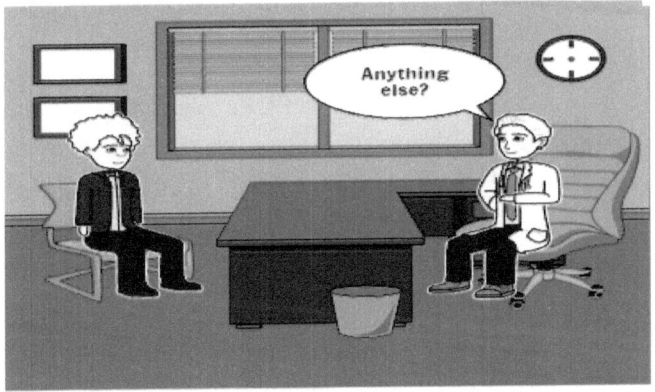

Aphorism 86:

"When the narrators have finished what they would say of their own accord, the physician then reverts to each particular symptom and elicits more precise information respecting it in the following manner; he reads over the symptoms as they were related to him one by one, and about each of them he inquires for further

particulars, e.g., at what period did this symptom occur? Was it previous to taking the medicine he had hitherto been using? While taking the medicine? Or only some days after leaving off the medicine? What kind of pain, what sensation exactly, was it that occurred on this spot? Where was the precise spot? Did the pain occur in fits and by itself, at various times? Or was it continued, without intermission? How long did it last? At what time of the day or night, and in what position of the body was it worst, or ceased entirely? What was the exact nature of this or that event or circumstance mentioned – described in plain words?"

Once the patinet has finished narrating all his complaints the physician shall go back to enquire in detail about each of those complaints to ensure that they are complete with respect to their modalities and other pecularities. An attempt should be made to complete each symptom with respect to its loaction, sensation, modalities, onset etc by skillfull questioning that ensures a smooth flow of conversation.

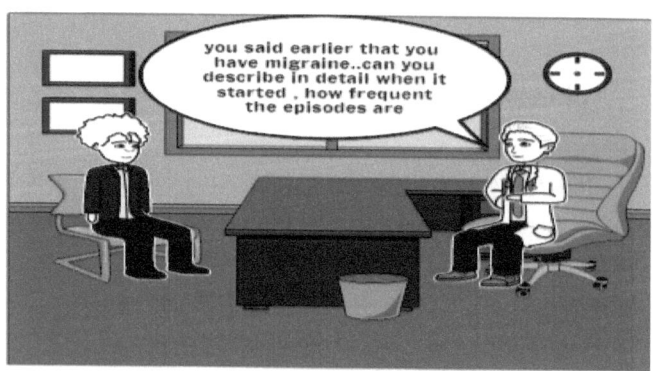

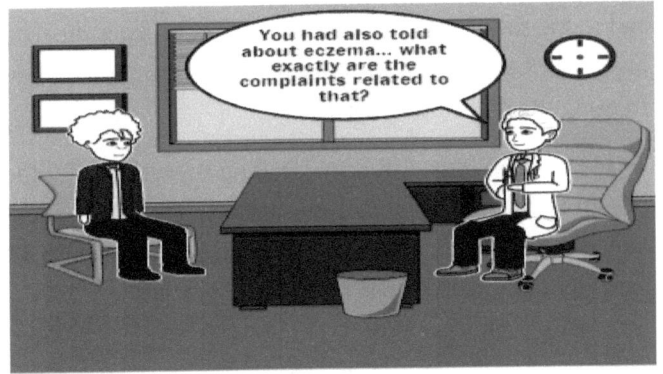

Aphorism 87:

"And thus the physician obtains more precise information respecting each particular detail, but without ever framing his questions so as to suggest the answer to the patient1, so that he shall only have to answer yes or no; else he will be misled to answer in the affirmative or negative something untrue, half true, or not strictly correct, either from indolence or in order to please his interrogator, from which a false picture of the disease and an unsuitable mode of treatment must result."

1 For instance the physician should not ask, Was not this or that circumstance present? He should never be guilty of making such suggestions, which tend to seduce the patient into giving a false answer and a false account of his symptoms.

Framing the questions is also an intergral part of case taking. The questions should be framed in such a way that it shall not disturb the continuity of communication and at the same time the flow of discussion goes on. The physician has to keep in mind certain precautions while framing the questions like:

He should not ask any leading questions ie the question that suggests answers because then the patient may give answers that shall not be reliable, false or partially true, hence misleading the physician.

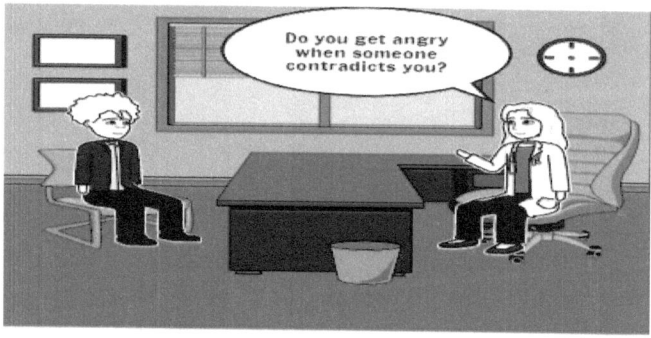

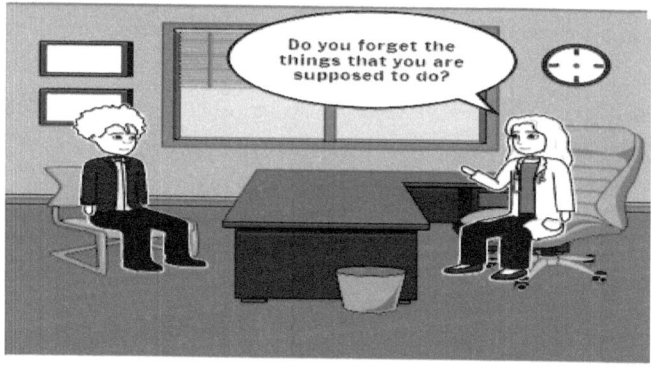

A physician should avoid asking direct questions for which the patient may answer neither an "yes" or a "No". Questions should be framed in such a way that the patient has to elaborate the answer.

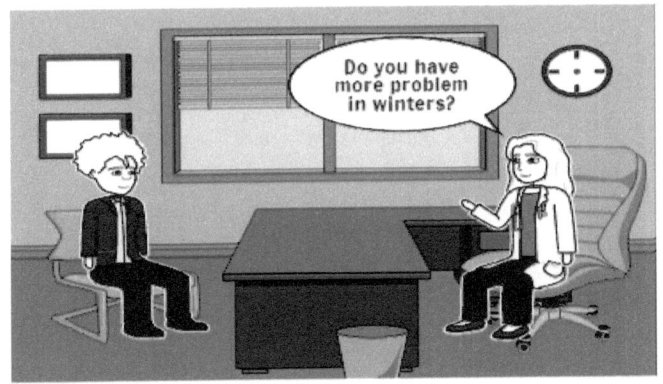

Wrong approach

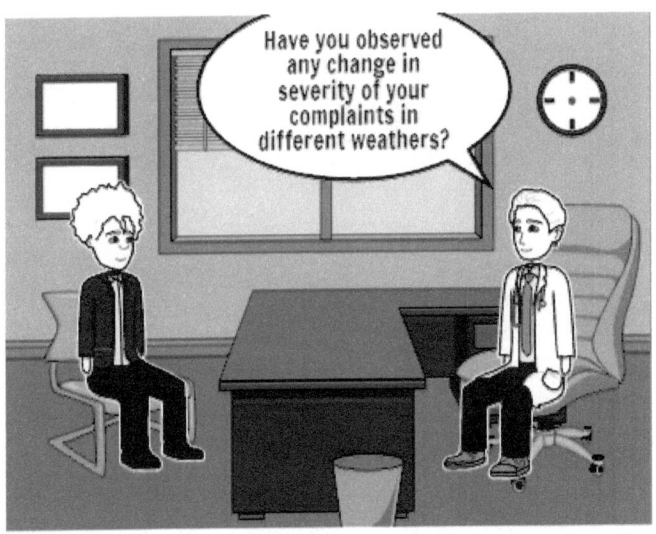

Right approach

The physician should not ask multiple choice questions because then the patient may choose an option randomly which may not be true or partially true.

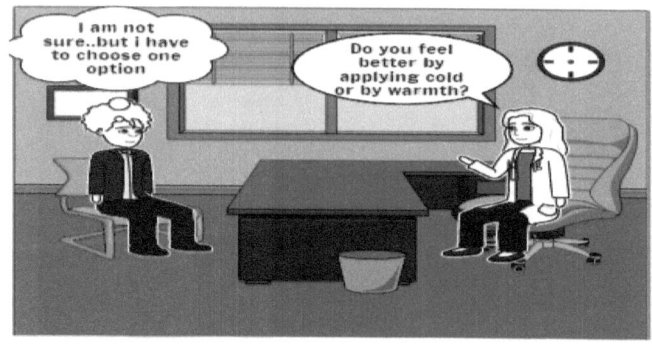

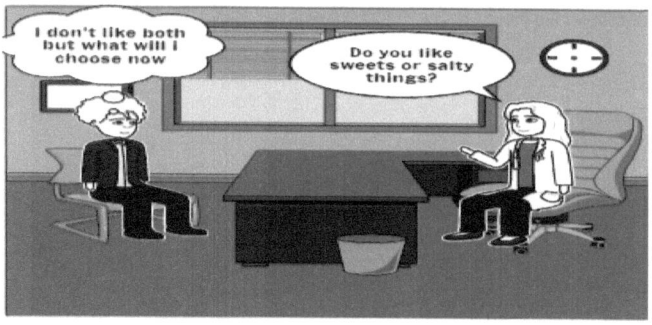

Aphorism 88:

"If in these voluntary details nothing has been mentioned respecting several parts or functions of the body or his metal state, the physician asks what more can be told in regard to these parts and these functions, or the state of his disposition or mind1, but in doing this he only makes use of general expressions, in order that his informants may be obliged to enter into special details concerning them."

1 For example what was the character of his stools? How does he pass his water? How is it with his day and night sleep? What is the state of his disposition, his humor, his memory? How about the thirst? What

sort of taste has he in his mouth? What kinds of food and drink are most relished? What are most repugnant to him? Has each its full natural taste, or some other unusual taste? How does he feel after eating or drinking? Has he anything to tell about the head, the limbs or the abdomen?

Usually during a skillfull case taking the physician shall get all those information both at mental level and physical level that he needs to construct the totality. However, if once the patient has finished narrating his complaints in order to trace out the complete picture the physician may have to ask certain questions in regarding to the parts affected and their functions. While doing so he also has to ensure that he is not putting in words into the patients mouth.

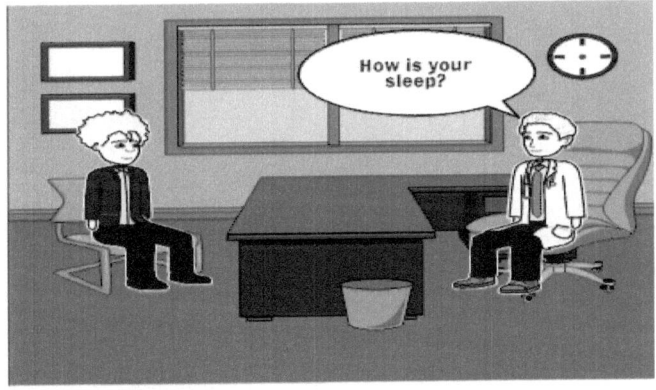

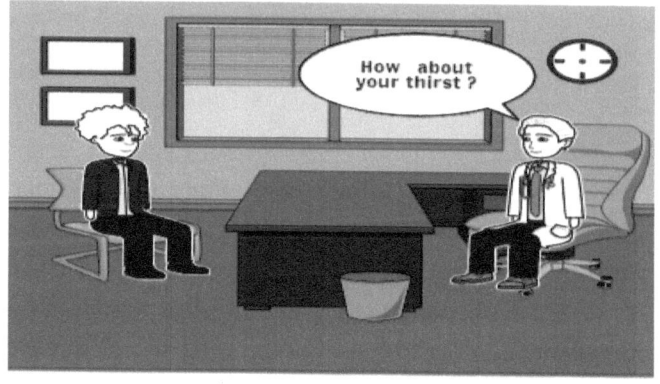

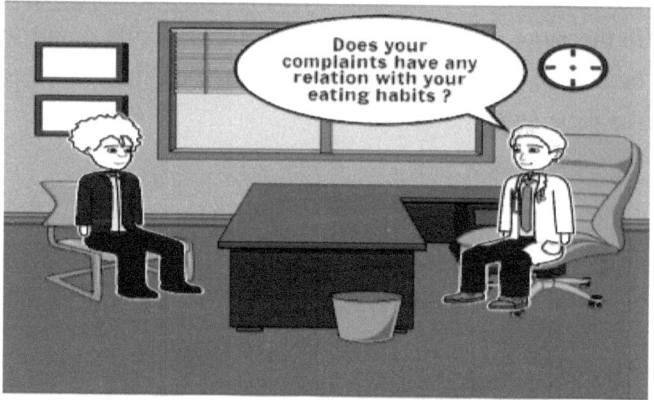

We all understand the importance of mental symptoms but clinically majority of us find it difficult to trace the mental symptoms. Usually patients are not aware of what we need from them to make a sucessful prescription, so they tend to narrate only those information which they are used to narrating. Hence only through skillfull questioning we can trace out the mental dispostion of the patient.

In some cases, while they narrate their physical symptoms their mental disposition shall also get reflected but in order to trace those, one should pay careful attention to the statements being made by the patient. Here is an example:

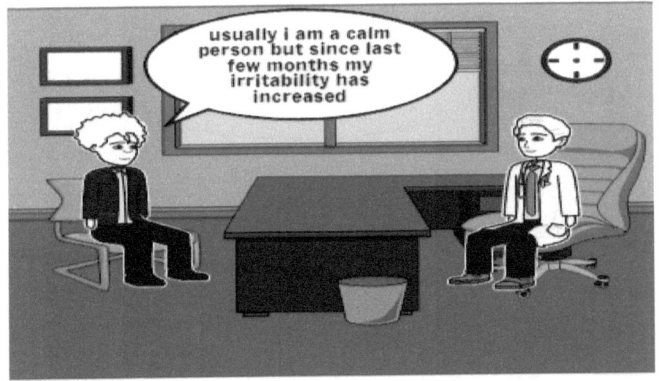

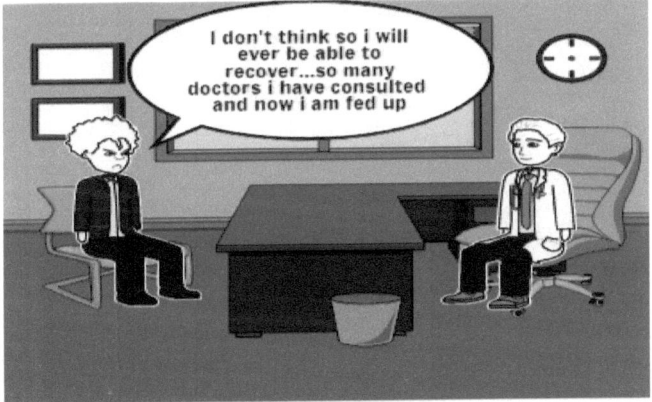

Altered irritability from the first image and despair of recovery from the second image above are the symptoms pertaining to mental plane.

In order to trace out the quality mental symptoms the physician should frame his questions in such a way that the impression should go to the patient as if the physician is interested, eager and curious to know the information he is asking for.

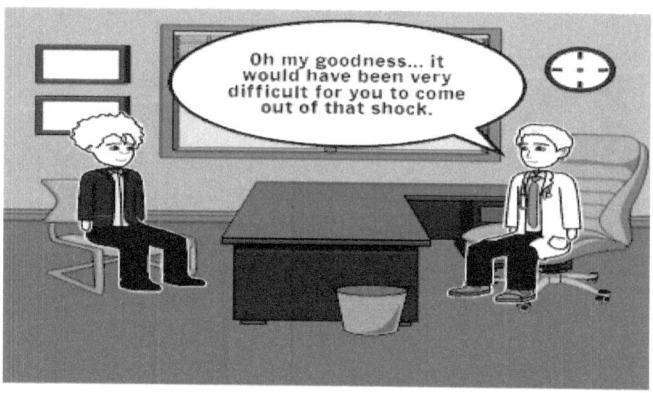

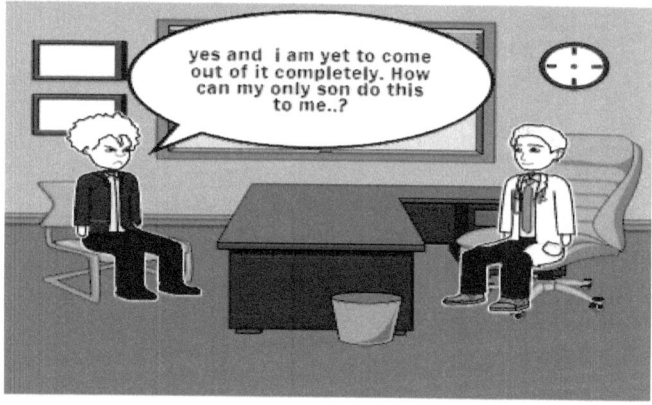

Aphorism 89:

"When the patient (for it is on him we have chiefly to rely for a description of his sensations, except in the case of feigned diseases) has by these details, given of his own accord and in answer to inquiries, furnished the

requisite information and traced a tolerably perfect picture of the disease, the physician is at liberty and obliged (if he feels he has not yet gained all the information he needs) to ask more precise, more special questions."

Once the patient has finished narrating all he has to tell the physician should be able to trace out the prefect image of the disease. But if he still feels that some more information may be required, he then has the liberty to ask more precise questions in order to complete the picture. However, he also has to ensure that he is not mounting any information upon the patient just for the sake of completing the picture.

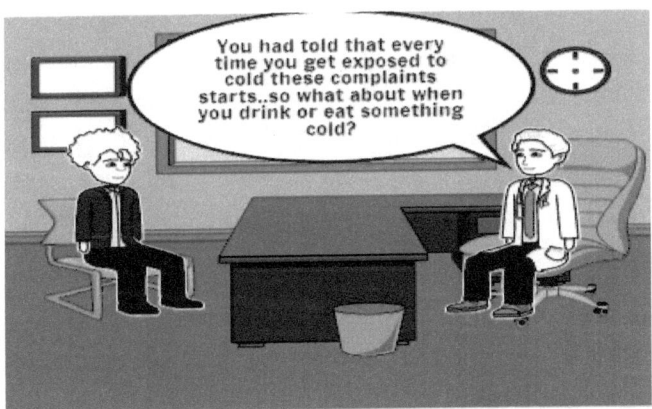

Aphorism 90:

"When the physician has finished writing down these particulars, he then makes a note of what he himself

observes in the patient, and ascertains how much of that was peculiar to the patient in his healthy state."

It has to be remembered that there are certain pecularities in an individual when he is healthy and pecularities identifies him as a seperate individual. These pecularities when group together forms the symptoms of normal disposition (Discussed in detail under classification of symptoms).

At the same in every individual there are certain pecularities that are induced in him as a result of the sickness. Such pecularities when grouped together forms the symptoms of altered or changed disposition.

Physician once done with the case taking has to now ascertain and classify the symptoms to separate the symptoms of normal disposition and changed disposition. The symptoms of altered or changed disposition has high value especially in acute cases provided they are very peculiar to the individual person.

The patient's facial expressions, way of answering, dullness, behaviour patterns etc has also to be studied carefully in order to differentiate the pecularities of altered disposition.

Aphorism 91:

"The symptoms and feelings of the patient during a previous course of medicine do not furnish the pure picture of the disease; but on the other hand, those

symptoms and ailments which he suffered from before the use of the medicines, or after they had been discontinued for several days, give the true fundamental idea of the original form of the disease, and these especially the physician must take note of. When the disease is of a chronic character, and the patient has been taking medicine up to the time he is seen, the physician may with advantage leave him some days quite without medicine, or in the meantime administer something of an unmedicinal nature and defer to a subsequent period the more precise scrutiny of the morbid symptoms, in order to be able to grasp in their purity the permanent uncontaminated symptoms of the old affection and to form a faithful picture of the disease."

Homoepathic remedy can be selected only after forming the true conceptual image of sickness (Discussed in detail in Chapter 2 of this book). This image can be formed only with the true symptoms of sickness that belongs to the patient. Most often especially in chronic diseases patients resort to homoepath only as their last option after having tried all other possible alternatives.

When a patient comes in such a state where he is either continuing a previous course of medicine or has taken lot of medicines in the past, the symptoms traced during the consultation may not reflect the true nature of disease and may present a set of modified or altered symptoms. Such symptoms does not reflect the true picture of disease. In such a situation the physician after taken into account the complete state of the case may advise the patient to discontinue the previous course of medicine and leave him for some days without giving any medicine or keep him on placebo and allow the true symptoms to appear again so that he may be in a position to construct the true image of sickness.

Palliative tretments has a limited span of action and when discontinued the orginal symptoms are bound to relapse. These set of orginal unmodified symptoms that is peculair to the given individual should form the base for constructing the totality.

In chronic cases the patients do not usually expect a miracle overnight but still it may be difficult for the physician to convince him to stop immediately all the previous medication and stay without any medicines. In such cases placebos can be given to the patient and convincing him logically why we do so. Many a times the facts have to be presented in a tactful way so that the trust and support the patient has build on the physician remains strong and the patient shall give enough time for the physician to raise the true nature of sickness.

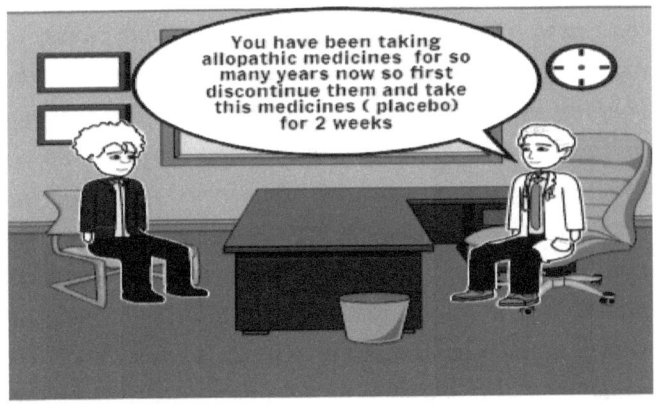

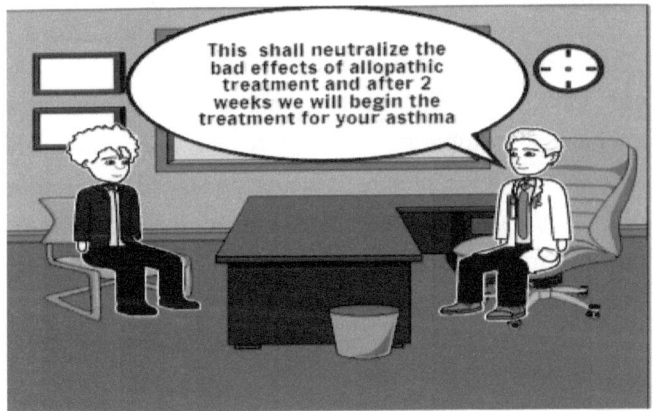

Aphorism 92:

"But if it be a disease of a rapid course, and if its serious character admit of no delay, the physician must content himself with observing the morbid condition, altered though it may be by medicines, if he cannot ascertain what symptoms were present before the employment of the medicines, – in order that he may at

least form a just apprehension of the complete picture of the disease in its actual condition, that is to say, of the conjoint malady formed by the medicinal and original diseases, which from the use of inappropriate drugs is generally more serious and dangerous than was the original disease, and hence demands prompt and efficient aid; and by thus tracing out the complete picture of the disease he will be enabled to combat it with a suitable homoeopathic remedy, so that the patient shall not fall a sacrifice to the injurious drugs he was swallowed."

In diseases of rapid course wherein the physician may not have enough time to wait and trace the true unchanged symptoms of disease he may take into account whatever picture is being presented at the time of consultation and a remedy can be admisnistered based on the totality formed out of the conjoint malady (medicinal + original diseases).

Aphorism 93:

"If the disease has been brought on a short time or, in the case of a chronic affection, a considerable time previously, by some obvious cause, then the patient – or his friends when questioned privately – will mention it either spontaneously or when carefully interrogated."

Causitive factor always plays a very important role in helping a physician to reach at the right remedy. In acute cases since the changes induced are very recent the patient or his by standers shall be able to spontaneoulsy specify it.

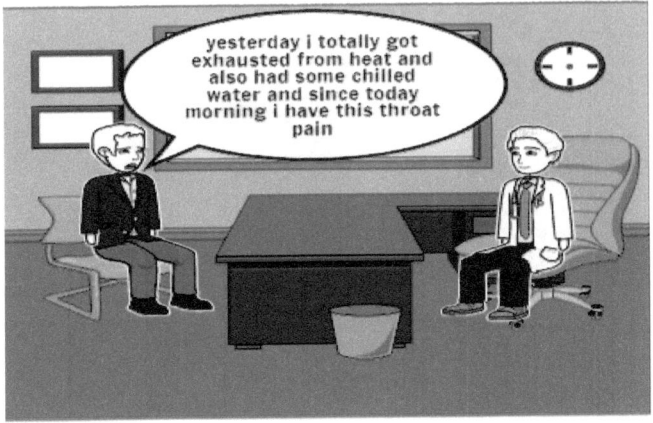

However, in some cases the patient himself may not be aware of as to what excatly the cause is for his acute illness. In such cases a careful interrogation into the activities of the patient few hours before the onset of illness may help the physician to identify the probable causitive factor.

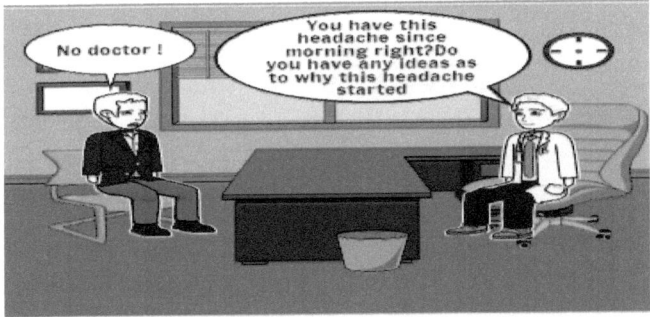

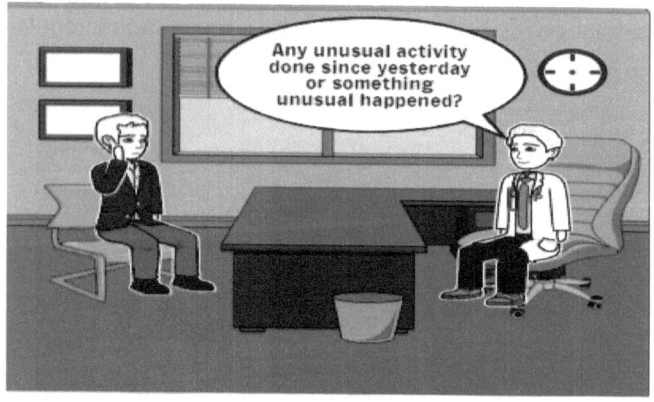

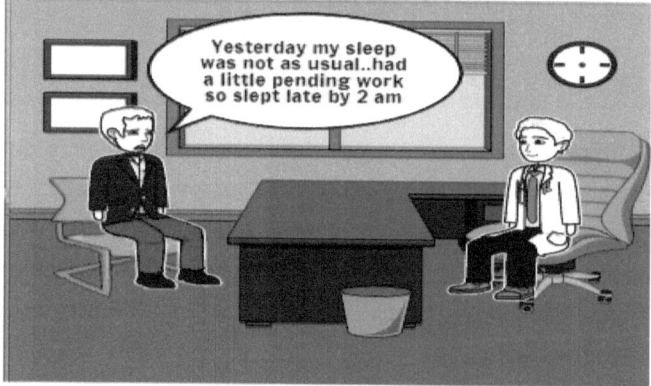

In chronic cases however the time period between the causitive factor affecting the person and the appearance of physical symptoms is quite long. The growth in such chronic cases happens at a very gradual pace so by the time the physical symptoms appear the patient may have forgotten the events that actually happened in his life at the time of onset. However even in such cases a detailed interrogation into all the impotant events from the patient's life few months before the actual appearance of initial symptoms shall help the physician to identify the probable cause.

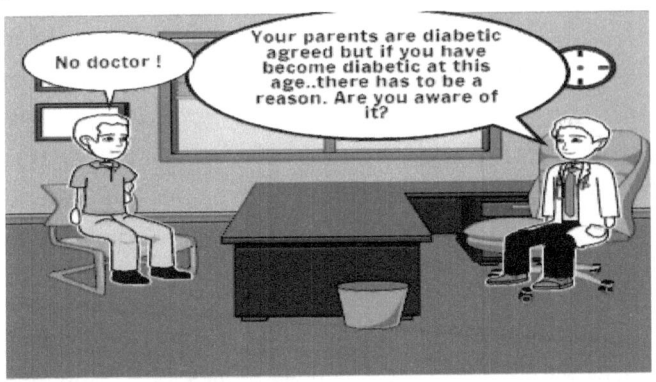

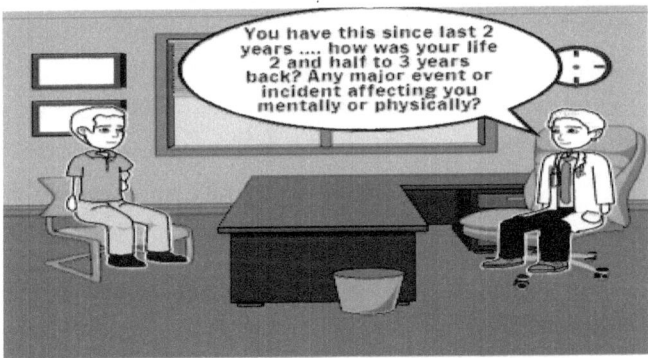

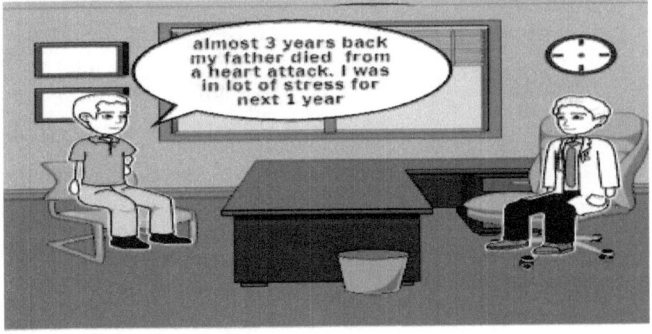

Aphorism 94:

"While inquiring into the state of chronic disease, the particular circumstances of the patient with regard to his ordinary occupations, his usual mode of living and diet, his domestic situation, and so forth, must be well considered and scrutinized, to ascertain what there is in them that may tend to produce or to maintain disease, in order that by their removal the recovery may by prompted"

It has to be kept in mind that for every individual there is a comfort zone which he defines for himself with respect to his occupation, mode of living, financial status, social status, dreams and expectations, diet, domestic situation etc. When a person lives under a condition which is within his comfort zone the chances are less that he may suffer from any derangement in health.

However, when a person is made to forced to live under any situation that goes outside his comfort zone then he basically starts compromising and this then invites diseases and also serve as a cause to maintain it.

While taking the case thus it becomes very improtant for a physician to understand deeply the occupation, mode of living, financial status, social status, dreams and expectations, diet, domestic situation etc., of the patient so that he can then judge as to what made the patient go out of his comfort zone and compromise with his living conditions. If any such factor exists in the persons life even at the time of consultation may act as a maintaining cause and if the same is able to be removed it shall then speed up the recovery process.

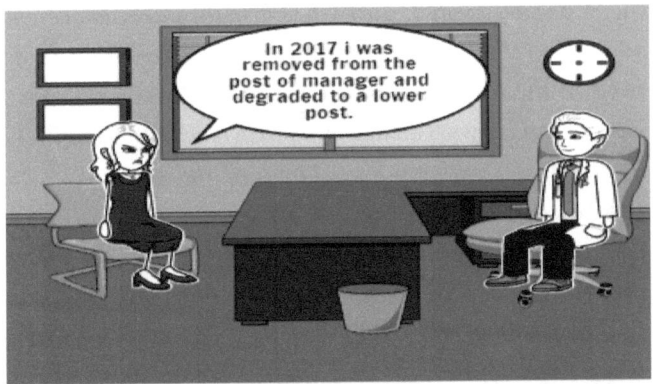

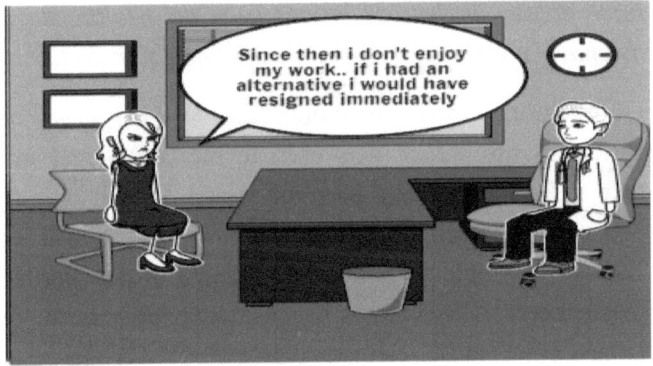

Aphorism 95:

"In chronic disease the investigation of the signs of disease above mentioned, and of all others, must be pursued as carefully and circumstantially as possible, and the most minute peculiarities must be attended to, partly because in these diseases they are the most

characteristic and least resemble those of acute diseases, and if a cure is to be affected they cannot be too accurately noted; partly because the patients become so used to their long sufferings that they pay little or no heed to the lesser accessory symptoms, which are often very pregnant with meaning (characteristic) – often very useful in determining the choice of the remedy – and regard them almost as a necessary part of their condition, almost as health, the real feeling of which they have well-nigh forgotten in the sometimes fifteen or twenty years of suffering, and they can scarcely bring themselves to believe that these accessory symptoms, these greater or less deviations from the healthy state, can have any connection with their principal malady."

In chronic cases sometimes due to long years of sufferings the patient gets used to the complaints and take it for granted as a part and parcel of their normal routine life. Such group of symptoms are called as accessory symptoms. Often the patients do not narrate these accessory symptoms because either they no more believe that those can be removed or due to long sufferings they tend to become used to it and adjust themselves in such a way that those complaints become a part of their routine life.

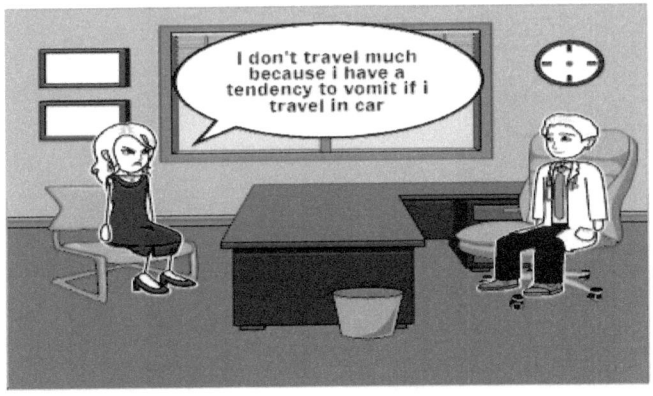
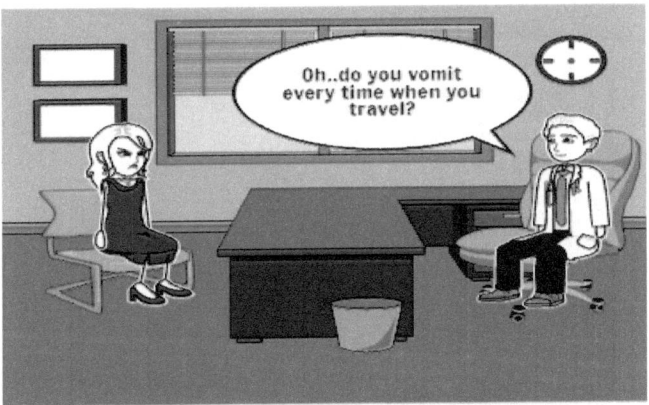
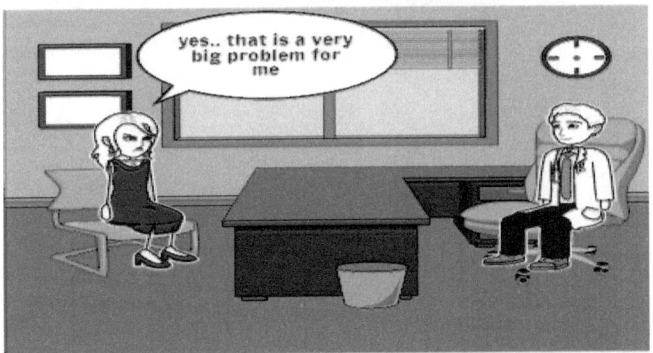

Step by step approach to practice classical homoeopathy

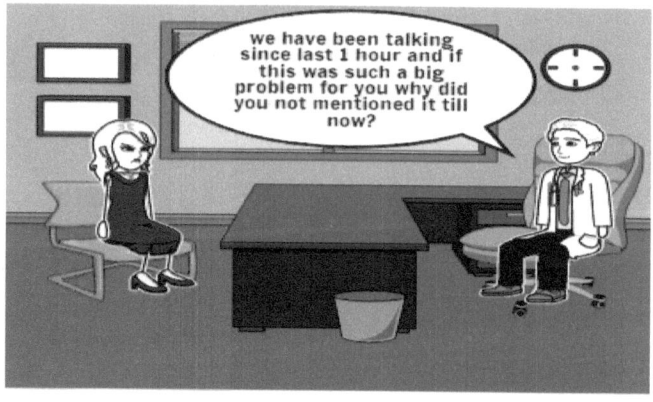

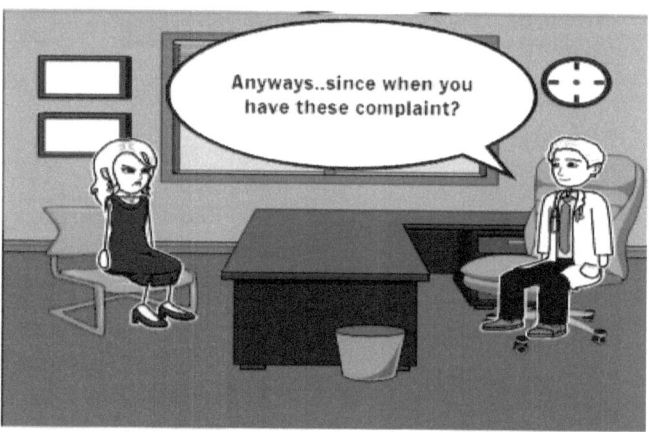

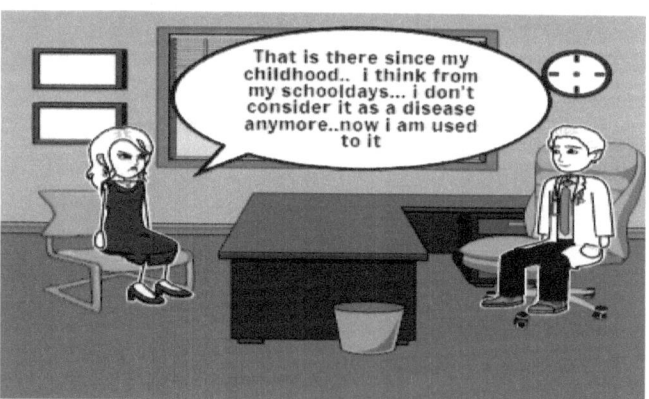

Such accessory symptoms are very important in forming the image of sickness. As mentioned usually patients do not reveal these until specifically asked. Hence only a through interrogation shall help to bring out such crutial informations.

Aphorism 96:

"Besides this, patients themselves differ so much in their dispositions, that some, especially the so-called hypochondriacs and other persons of great sensitiveness and impatient of suffering, portray their symptoms in too vivid colors and, in order to induce the physician to give them relief, describe their ailments in exaggerated expression"

The above aphorsim alerts the physician about the hypochondriacs and hypersensitive patients.

Hypochondriacs are those patients who have a morbid anxiety about their health. Such people present with an imaginary illness and because of their anxiety towards their health they tend to describe their sufferings or complaints in a exaggerated way. The location, severity and intensity of symptoms keeps on changing with respect to the way they tend to narrate it.

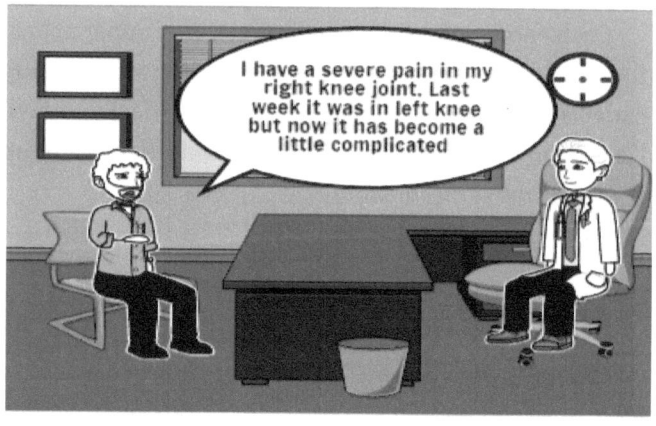

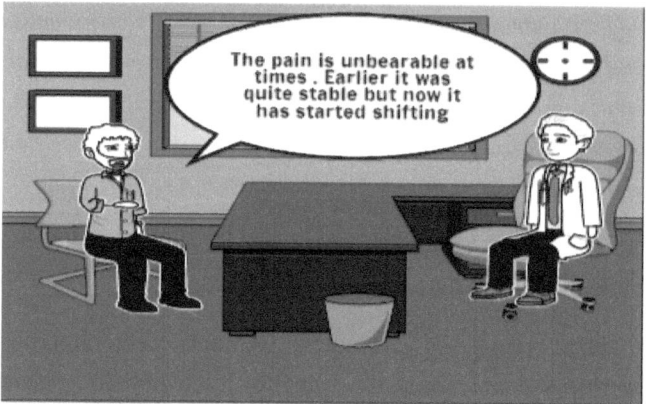

On the other hand, hypersesitives are those patients who generally exaggerate their sufferings. They describe their symptoms in such a way as if it has too much importance. Such people cannot tolerate a little suffering or pain. They tend to exaggerate to get more attention from the physician.

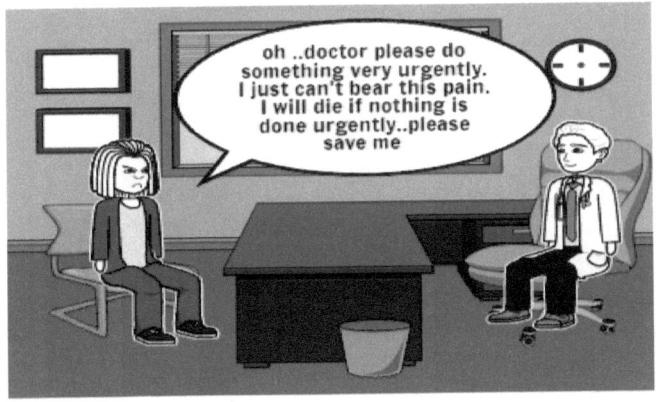

Aphorism 97:

"Other individuals of an opposite character, however, partly from indolence, partly from false modesty, partly from a kind of mildness of disposition or weakness of mind, refrain from mentioning a number of their symptoms, describe them in vague terms, or allege some of them to be of no consequence."

There are also some people who out of their laziness, lack of interest, mildness or false modesty do not describe their complaints in detail.

Step by step approach to practice classical homoeopathy

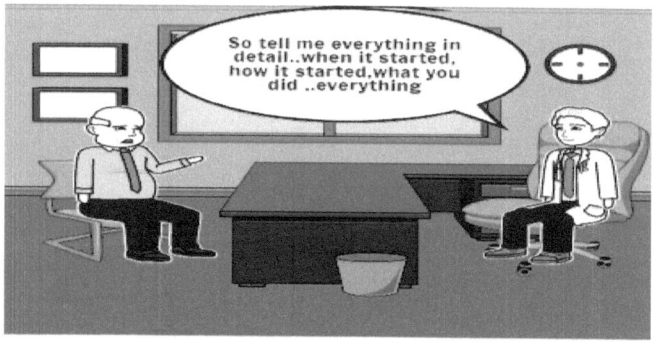

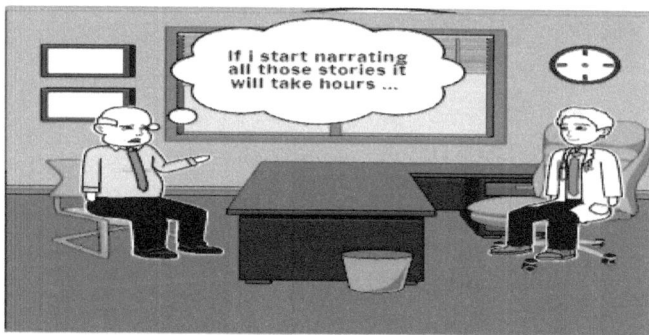

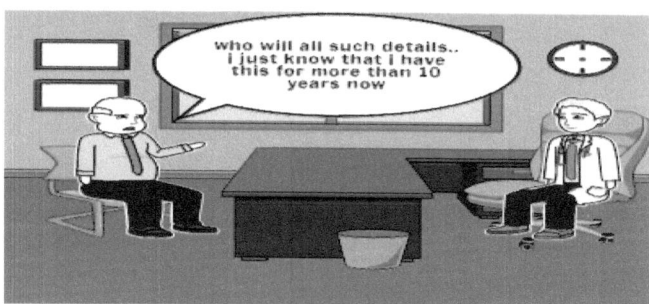

Indolence or laziness

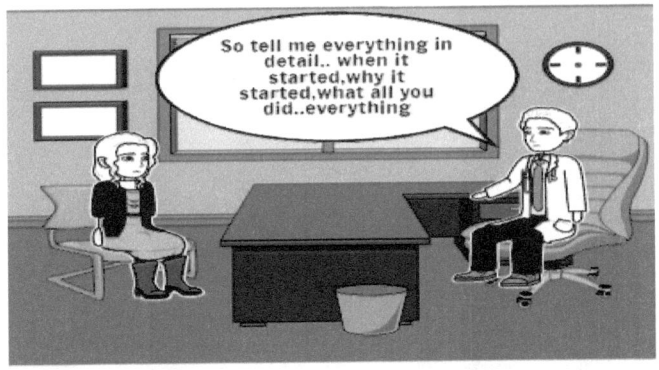

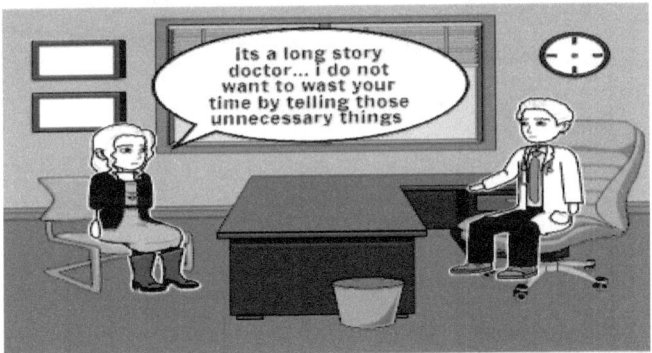

False modesty

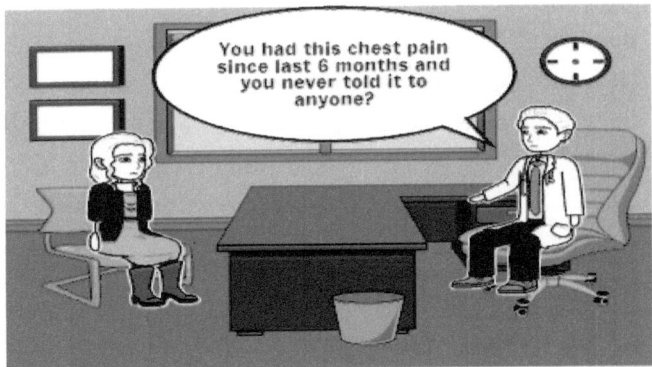

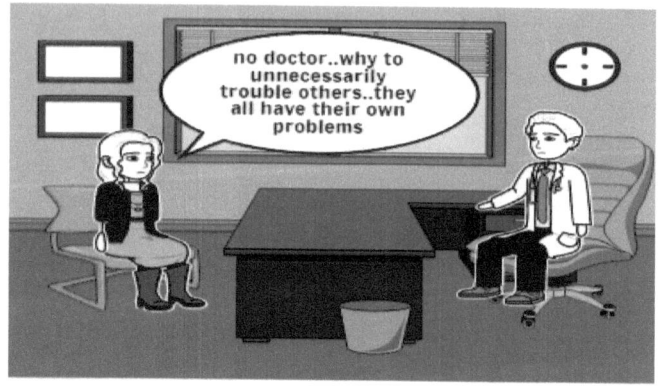

Mildness

Aphorism 98:

"Now, as certainly as we should listen particularly to the patient's description of his sufferings and sensations, and attach credence especially to his own expressions wherewith he endeavors to make us understand his ailments – because in the mouths of his friends and attendants they are usually altered and erroneously stated, – so certainly, on the other hand, in all diseases, but especially in the chronic ones, the investigation of the true, complete picture and its peculiarities demands especial circumspection, tact, knowledge of human nature, caution in conducting the inquiry and patience in an eminent degree."

A physician should give more priority and weightage to what the pateint is narratuing about himself and his complaints bacause the sensations and complaints can be descrinbed most accurately only by the patient himnself. Also, the intensity of symptoms and its modalities only the patient can feel and hence the most accurate information can be traced only from the patients mouth.

While taking a chronic case in order to tarce the true and complete picture a physician should posses the following qualities

a) <u>Especial circumspection</u>: Circumspection means the quality of being wary and unwilling to take risks; prudence. A physician should never take any risk to jump into any sort of conclusions without proper and careful observation of all the facts avialable that are peculiar to health and disease in that ndividual.

b) <u>Tact:</u> Tracking out required information from the patient is a tact. It involves tactful approach in handling the patient and framing the questions in an artistic way to ensure a smooth flow of communuication. The tact also includes perceiving the feelings and emotions of the patients so that after proper interpretation an accurate conclusion can be drawn regarding the mental plane of the person and the overall picture of his sufferings.

c) <u>Knowledge of human nature</u>: The physician should be aware of the normal feelings, common expected reactions and behavioural patterns of individuals under various conditions so that he can promptly trace if any devialtions are observed from the normal expected reaction or behaviour that shall indvidulaize the patient.

d) <u>Caution in conducting Inquiry</u>: The physician shall have to also ensure that while conducting the inquiry he does not hurt any feelings of the patient either intentionally or unintentionally. The care has to be taken while framing the questions especially with regards to something that is very persnal to the patient.

e) <u>Patience</u>: It's said that in homoepathy to get patients the physician needs to have patience. Not all patients develop that trust and confidence in the physician during the very first consultation. For some patients it takes time to come out with details that are very personal to them. A physician should always have that patience to wait for the patient to speak out openly and he should not force him for the same during the very first consulatation.

Aphorism 99:

"On the whole, the investigation of acute diseases, or of such as have existed but a short time, is much the easiest for the physician, because all the phenomena and deviations from the health that has been put recently lost are still fresh in the memory of the patient and his friends, still continue to be novel and striking. The physician certainly requires to know everything in such cases also; but he has much less to inquire into; they are for the most part spontaneously detailed to him".

Handling acute cases is comparitively easy for a physician than treating a chronic case because in acute cases all the deviations and alterations in the state of health are quite recent and the patients and his by standers shall promptly be able to describe all the changes in detail most ofte including its causitive factor which makes the task of a physician easy.

Aphorism 100:

"In investigating the totality of the symptoms of epidemic and sporadic diseases it is quite immaterial whether or not something similar has ever appeared in the world before under the same or any other name. The novelty or peculiarity of a disease of that kind makes no difference either in the mode of examining or of treating it, as the physician must any way regard to pure picture of every prevailing disease as if it were something new and unknown, and investigate it thoroughly for itself, if he desire to practice medicine in a real and radical manner, never substituting conjecture for actual observation, never taking for granted that the case of disease before him is already wholly or partially known, but always carefully examining it in all its phases; and this mode of procedure is all the more requisite in such cases, as a careful examination will show that every prevailing disease is in many respects a phenomenon of a unique character, differing vastly from all previous epidemics, to which certain names have been falsely applied – with the exception of those epidemics resulting

from a contagious principle that always remains the same, such as smallpox, measles, etc".

While handling epidemic and sporadic dieases the physician have to ensure that he carefully studies and examines each and every case and a individual one and not to get biased by his earlier exeriences of handling cases that may look similar. There has to be some individual pecularity associated with each and every such case that shall isolate it from other cases that may look similar in its form, existence and manifestations. The expections are those epidemics which are caused by the same source such as mallpox, measles etc.

Aphorism 101:

"It may easily happen that in the first case of an epidemic disease that presents itself to the physician's notice he does not at once obtain a knowledge of its complete picture, as it is only by a close observation of several cases of every such collective disease that he can become conversant with the totality of its signs and symptoms. The carefully observing physician can, however, from the examination of even the first and second patients, often arrive so nearly at a knowledge of the true state as to have in his mind a characteristic portrait of it, and even to succeed in finding a suitable, homoeopathically adapted remedy for it."

In epidemics the totality can be arrived at only after the physician makes a careful study of several cases to obtain the complete picture of the disease. However, if the physician is experienced enough having handled such situations before might get a complete picture by studying one or two cases of such epidemic outbreaks.

Aphorism 102:

"In the course of writing down the symptoms of several cases of this kind the sketch of the disease picture becomes ever more and more complete, not more spun out and verbose, but more significant (more characteristic), and including more of the peculiarities of this collective disease; on the one hand, the general symptoms (e.g., loss of appetite, sleeplessness, etc.) become precisely defined as to their peculiarities; and on the other, the more marked and special symptoms which are peculiar to but few diseases and of rarer occurrence, at least in the same combination, become prominent and constitute what is characteristic of this malady.1 All those affected with the disease prevailing at a given time have certainly contracted it from one and the same source and hence are suffering from the same disease; but the whole extent of such an epidemic disease and the totality of its symptoms (the knowledge whereof, which is essential for enabling us to choose the most suitable homoeopathic remedy for this array of symptoms, is obtained by a complete survey of the morbid picture) cannot be learned from one single patient, but is only to be perfectly deduced (abstracted)

and ascertained from the sufferings of several patients of different constitutions."

Only after a physician has studied carefully several cases, it would seen possible for him to get a clear and complete picture of the disease. The overall general symptoms and characteristic particulars has to be noted down seperately which then constitutes the totality of that epidemic. A remedy selected on the basis of this final totality is know as the "genus epidemicus" which can then be used as preventive and curative remedy for the given state of epidemic outbreak. It has to be very clearly kept in mind that genus epidemicus is not selected on the basis of the common particulars, but it is on the basis of overall general symptoms and characteristic particulars observed commonly after studing several cases during an epidemic outbreak.

Aphorism 103:

"In the same manner as has here been taught relative to the epidemic disease, which are generally of an acute character, the miasmatic chronic maladies, which, as I have shown, always remain the same in their essential nature, especially the psora, must be investigated, as to the whole sphere of their symptoms, in a much more minute manner than has ever been done before, for in them also one patient only exhibits a portion of their symptoms, a second, a third, and so on, present some other symptoms, which also are but a (dissevered, as it were), portion of the totality of the symptoms which

constitute the entire extent of this malady, so that the whole array of the symptoms belonging to such a miasmatic, chronic disease, and especially to the psora, can only be ascertained from the observation of very many single patients affected with such a chronic disease, and without a complete survey and collective picture of these symptoms the medicines capable of curing the whole malady homoeopathically (to wit, the antipsorics) cannot be discovered; and these medicines are, at the same time, the true remedies of the several patients suffering from such chronic affections."

Similarly, in chronic cases the maismatic expressions cannot be studied in a single person as it shall then yeild only partial expressions. When fundamental maisms affecting several people are studied individually and the partial pictures are logically combined that would form the complete picture of chronic miasmatic disease. An anti maismatic remedy is selected on the bais of such a totality would help several people suffering from these miasmatic diseases.

Aphorism 104:

"When the totality of the symptoms that specially mark and distinguish the case of disease or, in other words, when the picture of the disease, whatever be its kind, is once accurately sketched,1 the most difficult part of the task is accomplished. The physician has then the picture of the disease, especially if it be a chronic one, always before him to guide him in his treatment; he can

investigate it in all its parts and can pick out the characteristic symptoms, in order to oppose to these, that is to say, to the whole malady itself, a very similar artificial morbific force, in the shape of a homoeopathically chosen medicinal substance, selected from the lists of symptoms of all the medicines whose pure effects have been ascertained. And when, during the treatment, he wishes to ascertain what has been the effect of the medicine, and what change has taken place in the patient's state, at this fresh examination of the patient he only needs to strike out of the list of the symptoms noted down at the first visit those that have become ameliorated, to mark what still remain, and add any new symptoms that may have supervened."

Once is case taking is completed the physician now forms the image of sickness by logically rearranging the peculair and characteristic symptoms of the case. This image is then matched with a most similar image reflected by the remedy thereby the remedy shall fit in as the similimum for the given case. During the follow up all the changes both at physical level and mental plane has to be carefully noted down as long as the remedy shall continue to act.

Incase a new remedy needs to be selected after the first indicated remedy has served its purpose completely, the case has to be taken again considering it as a fresh case and a totality has to be formed based on the existing symptoms to construct a new conceptual image of sickness and accordingly a new remedy may be selected.

5. Classification of symptoms

Once we are done with case taking, we shall be left out with plenty of symptoms to work with. It has to be kept in mind that all observed symptoms in a case are not equally important. So, our next task is to give value to an observed symptom. For giving this value to each and every observed symptom it's very important for us to understand the classification of symptoms.

Symptoms can be broadly classified into two categories

- Symptoms of the patient
- Symptoms of the disease

Symptoms of the patient and symptoms of the disease originate from two different sources. We had discussed earlier as to how the disturbance strikes at the centre which then creates an imbalance that flows from the centre to the periphery affecting first our will and emotions. The individual tends to respond and react to this flow of imbalance in their own peculiar manner giving rise to the mental symptoms at emotional level (Altered disposition - discussed in detail later).

Similarly, as the imbalance affects the understanding and intellectual level it then gives rise to altered mental symptoms at intellectual or understanding level. Then the physical generalities are altered and finally when the physical symptoms appear on the materialistic level there also an individual reaction is shown at the particular level that give rise to the characteristic particulars. These characteristic particulars may be in the form of specific modalities (not a part of disease symptom) or specific concomitants.

On the other hand, when the imbalance finally gets settled or localized on a particular part (or parts) those part(s) then becomes vulnerable. It may also provide a soil for the growth of microbes or any other morbific agents which then interferes with the normal functioning of the bodily activities either generally or concerned with that affected part giving rise to yet another group of physical symptoms that we call the symptoms of the disease(see below illustration)

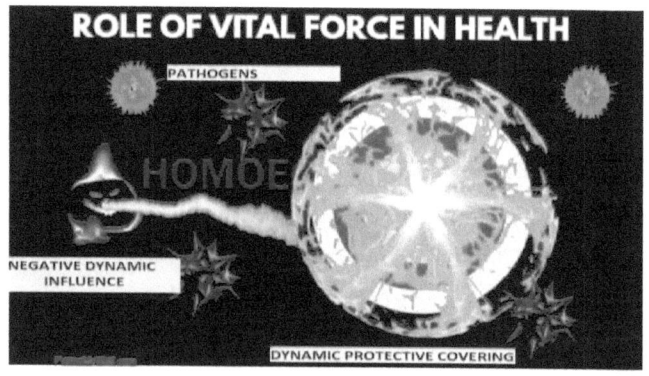

Figure 1

When the vital force is in order (Figure 1) the dynamic protective covering prevents the external negative dynamic influence to act upon the vital force and it also ensures that the external morbific agents (Pathogens) are not allowed to enter (self protection) the body.

If by any means such pathogens gains entry into the body the vital force when in order ensures that such pathogens are either killed or removed before they could cause any damage or destruction (self preservation).

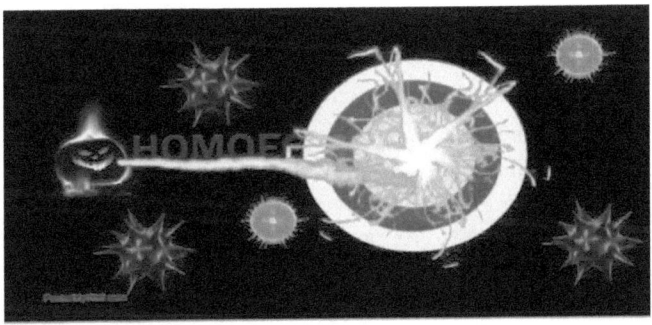

Figure 2

When the dynamic protective covering becomes weak the external negative dynamic influence is allowed to act upon the vital force causing its derangement. This derangement creates an imbalance which tends to flow from the centre to the periphery affecting first our will and emotions giving rise to the mental symptoms of altered disposition at emotional level. (Figure 3)

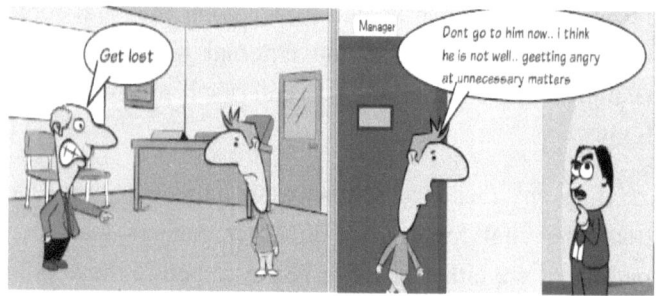

Figure 3

Then the understanding and intellect is affected giving rise to altered mental symptoms at intellectual level. (Figure 4)

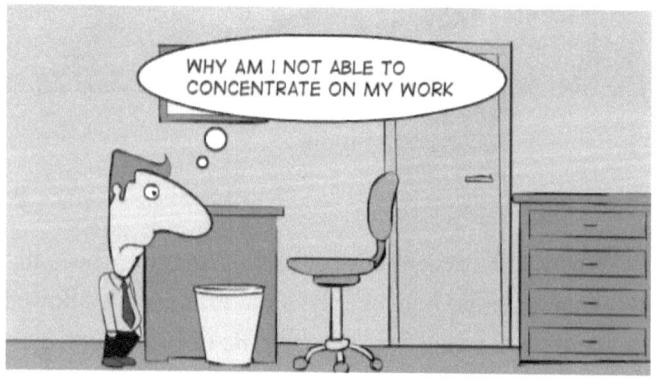

Figure 4

Then the physical generalities are altered. (Figure 5)

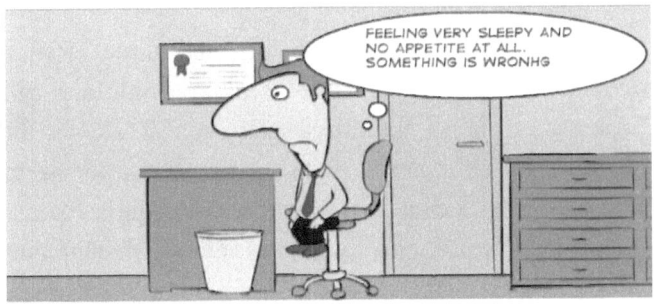

Figure 5

Finally, the physical symptoms appear at the materialistic plane. Here also we find certain individualistic peculiarities which constitutes the characteristic particulars. (Figure 6)

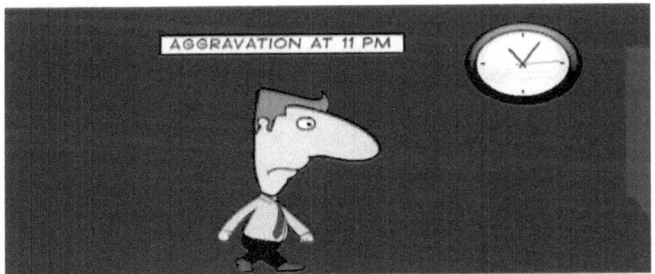

Figure 6

Ideally this symptom at individual level denotes the peculiarity of that person in reacting towards any disturbance. Such observed symptoms both at mental and physical level are grouped together to construct the totality of the case.

On the other hand when the vital force is in a deranged state its functions of self protection and self preservation is compromised and then it allows the negative morbific agents (both internal and external) to flourish at the localized part where the disturbance has got settled in causing to produce certain set of symptoms which we group together as the symptoms of the disease.

These symptoms of the disease are those common symptoms on the basis of which a clinical diagnosis is made. Such group of symptoms are common to all suffering from the disease having the same clinical diagnosis. (Figure 7)

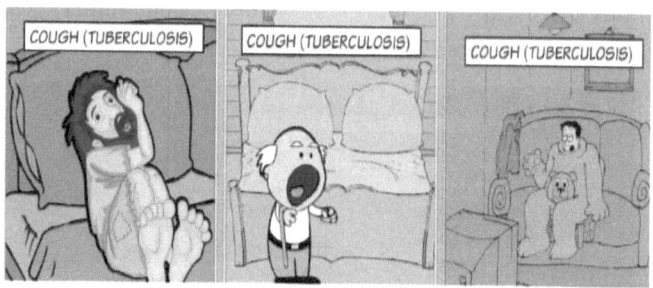

Figure 7

As you can see above that cough is a common symptom of the disease in patients having tuberculosis. These symptoms common to the diase have no role in selecting the homoeopathic remedy. A homoeopathic remedy has to be selected based on the individual peculiarities both at mental and physical level which we call it as the symptoms of the patient.

It has to be remembered that when a common symptom of the disease is accompanied by any specific modality or concomitant it then becomes the symptoms of the patient. The modality or concomitant has to be very specific uncommon and characteristic for this to apply. For example in figure 7 cough is a common symptom of the disease but in the first image the cough is aggravated when lying. Now this lying while aggravation is a common modality as in patients with tuberculosis the alveolar surface area available for gaseous exchange is compromised and while lying the cough is bound to increase. So here although the common symptom of cough is accompanied by a modality still it remains the common symptom of disease as the modality here is not specific peculiar and characteristic.

On the other hand, in second and third image you can see that there is aggravation while standing and sitting which is very specific peculiar and characteristic. Such modalities when accompanied with the common symptom of the disease then make it a characteristic symptom.

So far we have seen that symptoms can be broadly classified into two categories. Symptoms of the disease and symptoms of the patient. Symptoms of the disease shall help us to arrive at a precise clinical diagnosis whereas the symptoms of the patient help us to construct the totality.

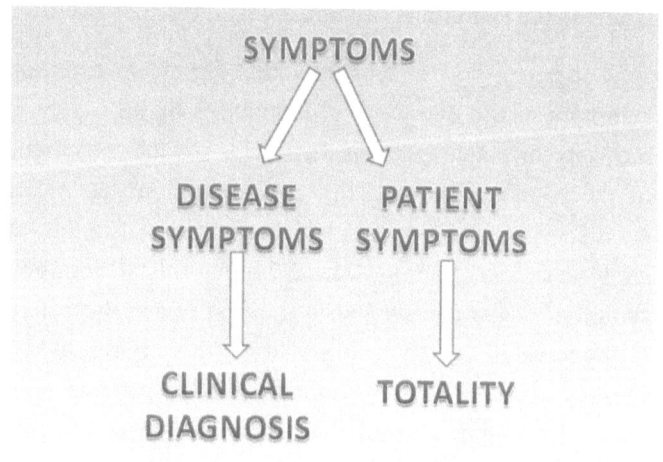

The observed symptoms can further be classified into two categories. It can either be a general symptom or particular symptoms.

General Symptoms

General symptoms are those symptoms which belong to the patient as a whole and are not related to any particular part of the body. They are further divided into two categories

- ➢ Mental generals
- ➢ Physical generals

Mental generals are those symptoms which belong to the patient as a whole at mental level. They are of two types

- ➢ Symptoms related to will and emotions
- ➢ Symptoms related to intellect and understanding

Examples of symptoms related to will and emotions

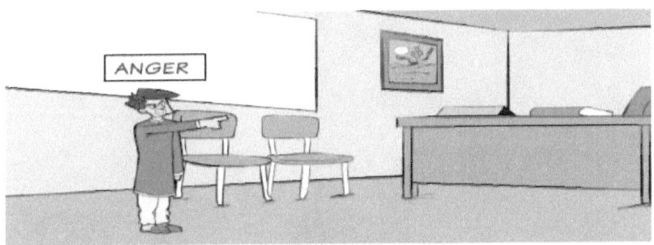

Anger

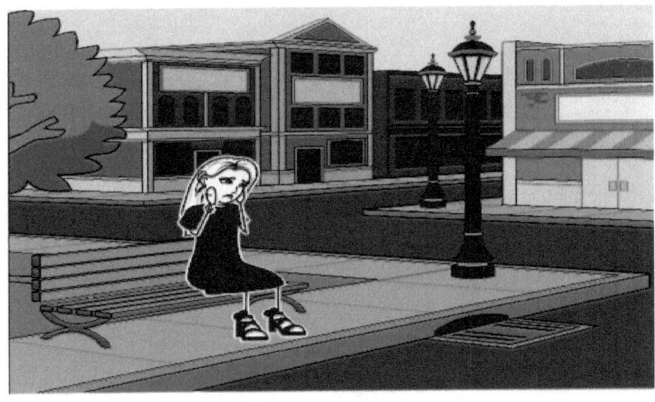

Sadness

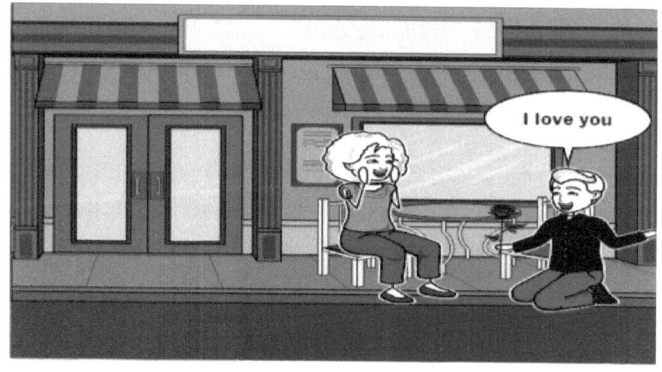

Love

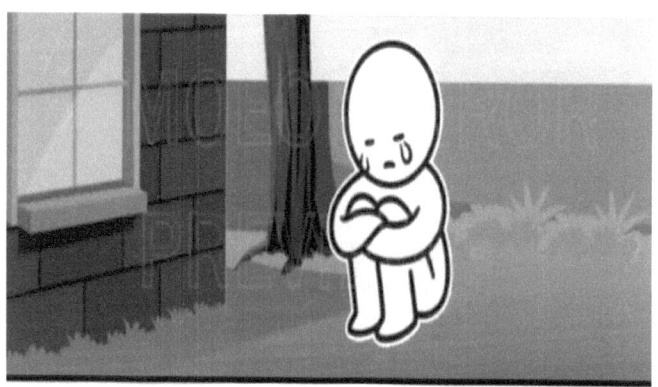

Weeping

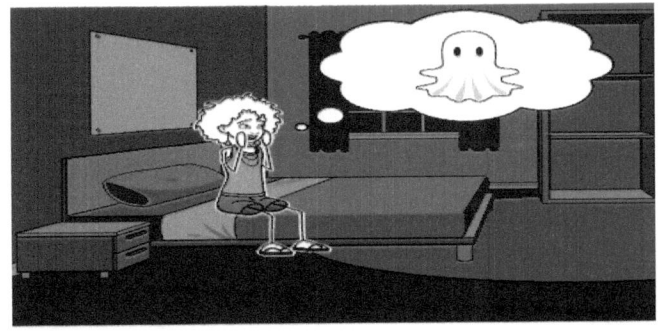

Fear

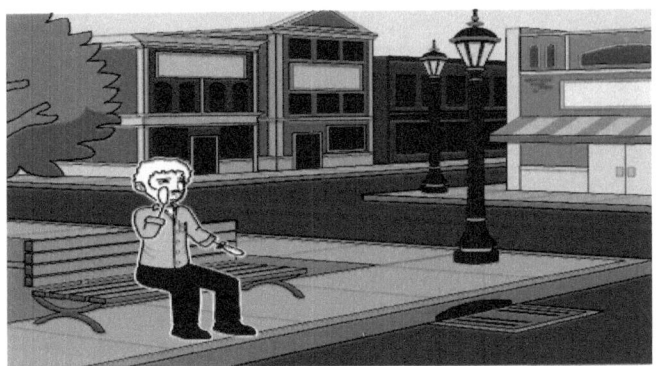

Depression, anxiety, panic or tension

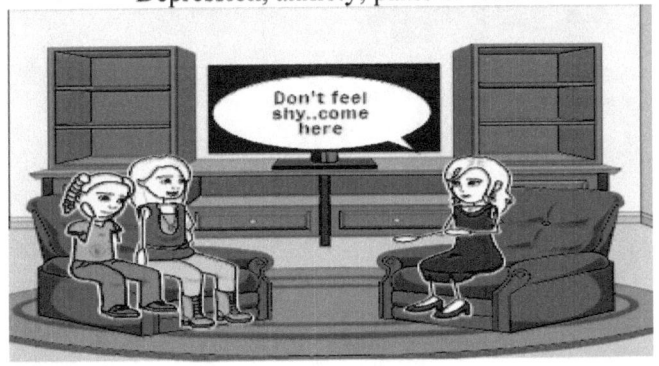

Shyness

In general, all symptoms related to any kind of feeling or emotions and categorized as mental generals at emotional level.

Examples of symptoms related to understanding and intellect includes

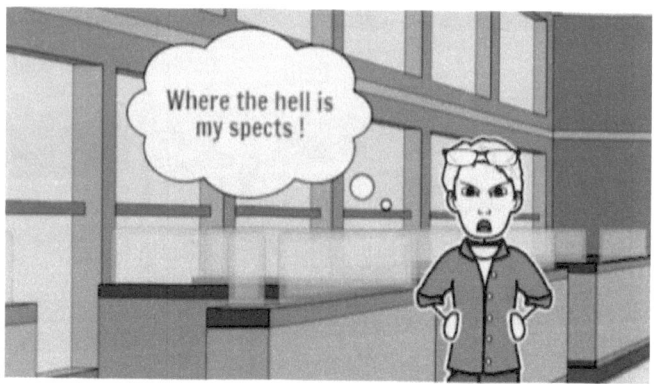

Absent minded

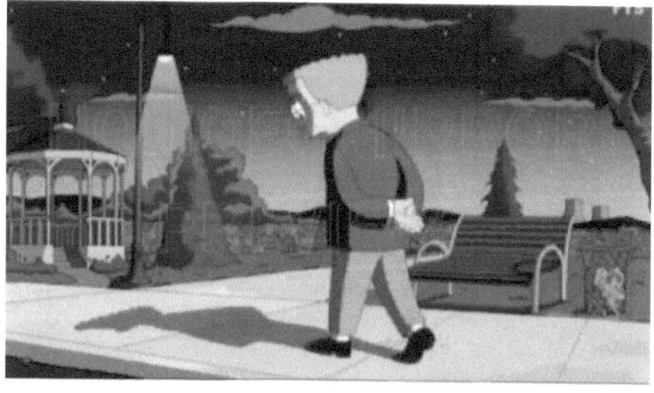

Impatience

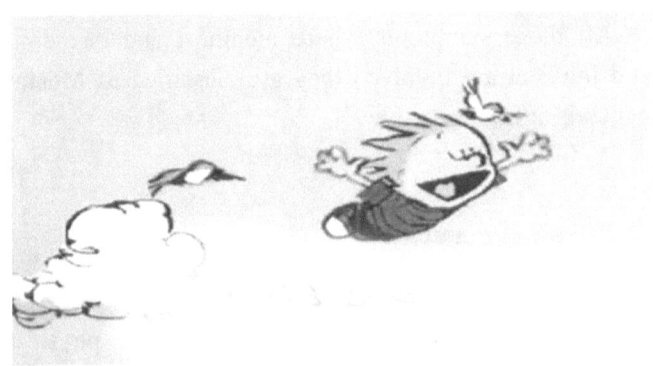

Illusion, delusions and hallucinations

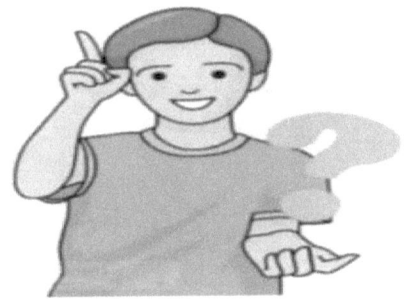

Memory

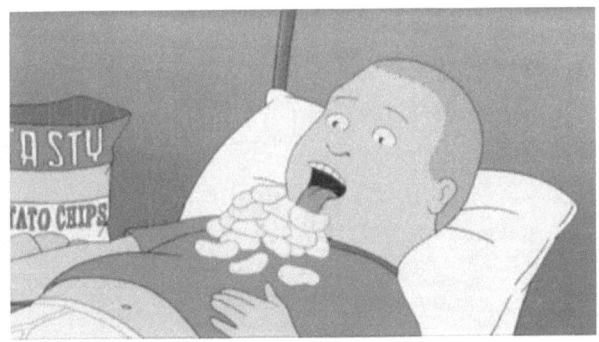

Laziness

All those symptoms where memory, understanding and intellect are involved they are classified as Mental generals at Intellectual level.

Physical generals

All those symptoms which are related to the person as a whole at physical level are called the physical generals. They include symptoms related to

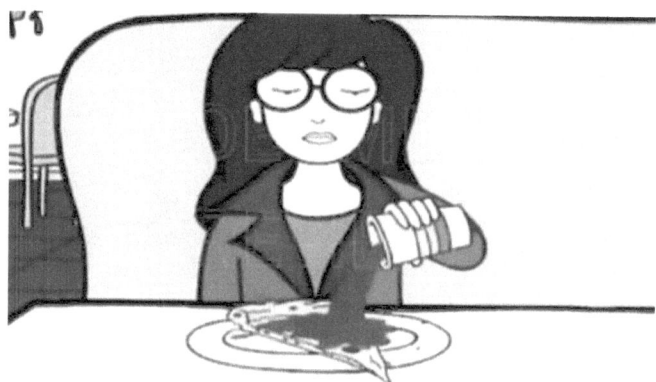

Appetite

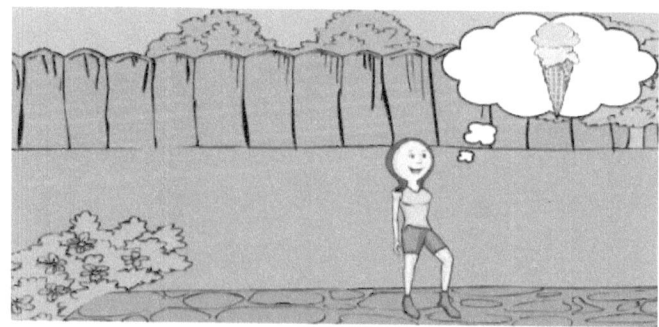

Desires & Avesions

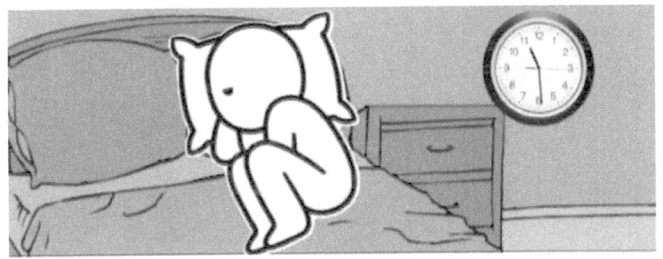

Sleep

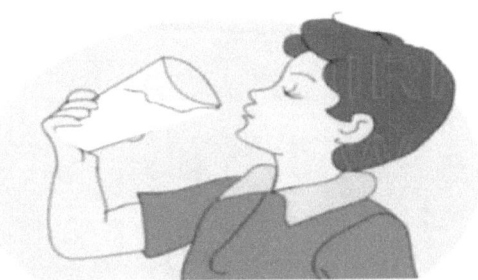

Thirst

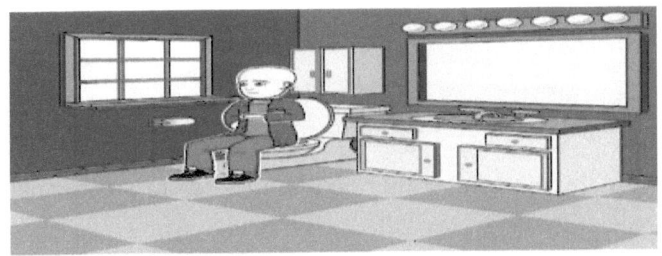

Bowel habirs & Urination

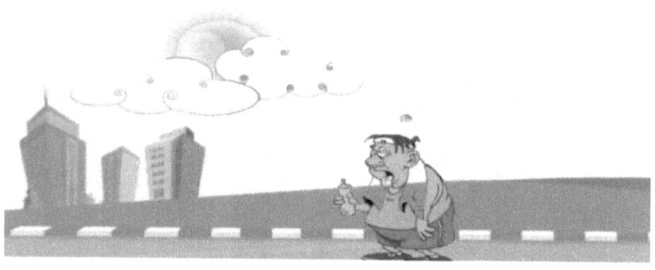

Prespiration

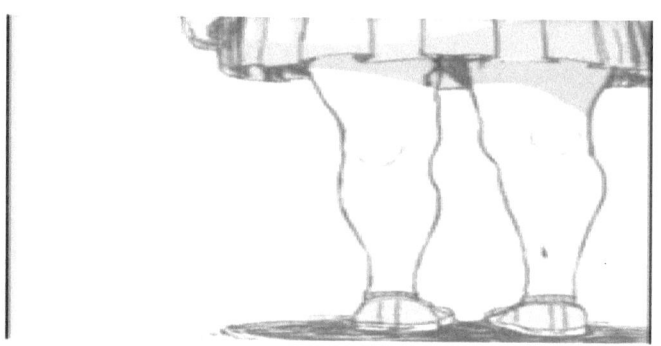

Symptoms related to menstruartion

Particular symptoms

All those symptoms which are related to a particular part of the body are called as particular symptoms. They represent the symptoms that appear after the imbalance flowing from centre to periphery gets localized on the materialistic plane. They are further divided into two

- Common particulars
- Characteristic particulars

Common particulars are those set of common symptoms that is found in all or majority of people suffering from the same disease. They are least important for the selection of a homoeopathic remedy and can be grouped together to reach at the precise clinical diagnosis. Some examples of common particulars are:

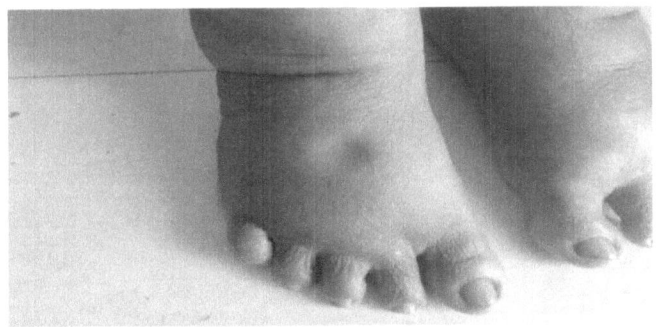

Pitting Oedema in cases of renal failure

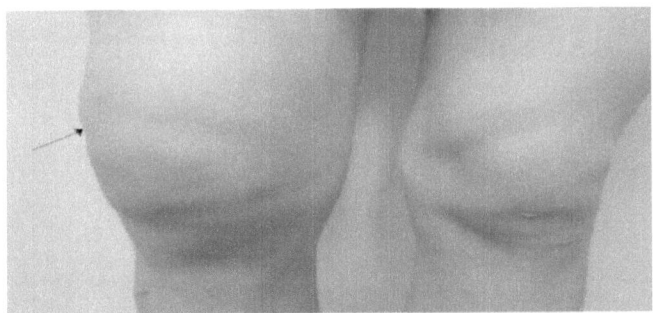

Swelling in cases of Arthritis

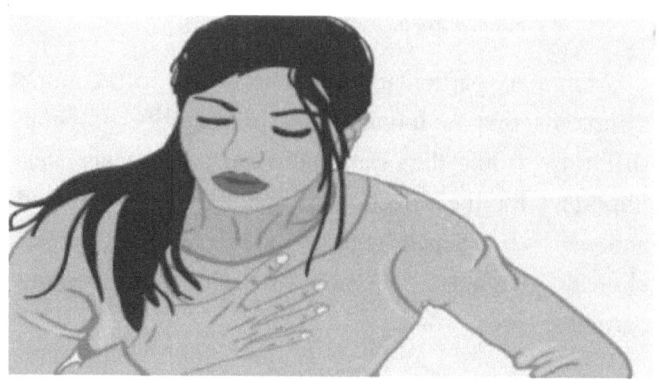

Breathing difficulty in asthma

Characteristic particulars are those which although remain localized to a certain part but still will be very striking and peculiar in that given case. Such symptoms are specific to the patient in particular and not common to any disease. Some of the examples of characteristic particulars are:

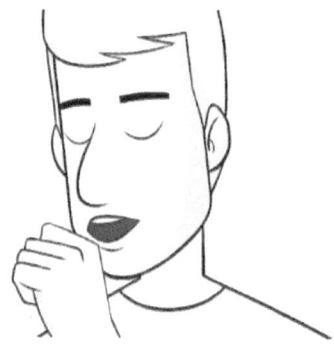

Hawking

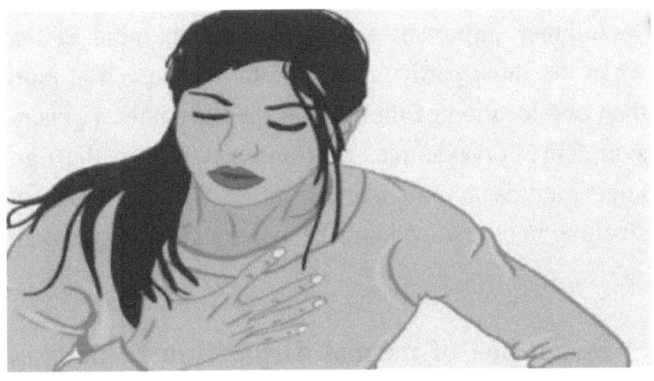

Breathing difficulty in asthma aggravated at 2 am

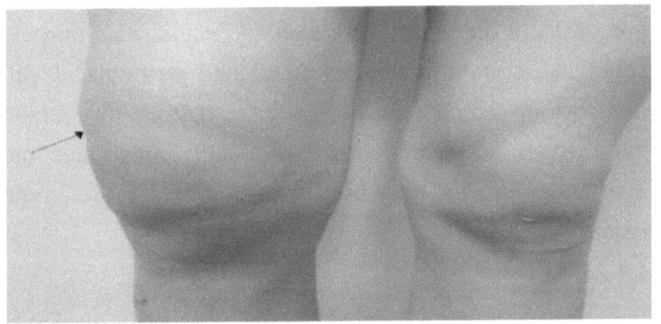

Swelling in arthrits ameliorated by walking

Characteristic particular symptoms are those symptoms which are unexpected to be present or is very peculiar and strange to a particular individual and not common to the disease. It has to be kept in mind that when a common particular is accompanied by a very specific strange modality or concomitant it then becomes a characteristic particular.

Another important aspect to keep in mind is that when the same particular symptom is observed at more than one location of the body it then becomes a general symptom. For example, pain and swelling in the right knee joint is a particular symptom whereas pain and swelling in both knee joints becomes a general symptom.

Symptoms of normal disposition & changed disposition

In each and every individual there are always a certain set of peculiarities found which isolate's that person from the other. These set of peculiarities may be found both at both general level and particular level. Such group of peculiarities which exists in the person even when he is in a state of health constitutes the symptoms of his normal disposition. Here are some examples:

Symptoms of normal disposition at mental level

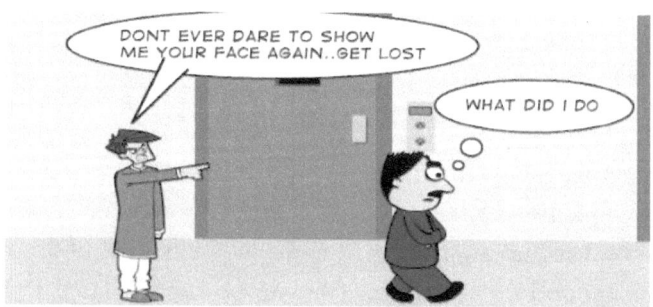

Easily getting angry (Mental symptom emotional level)

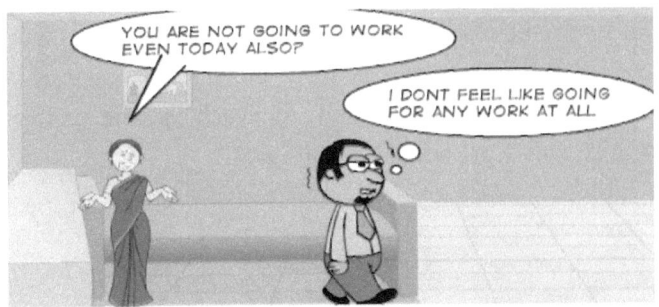

Laziness (Mental symptom - normal disposition - intellectual level)

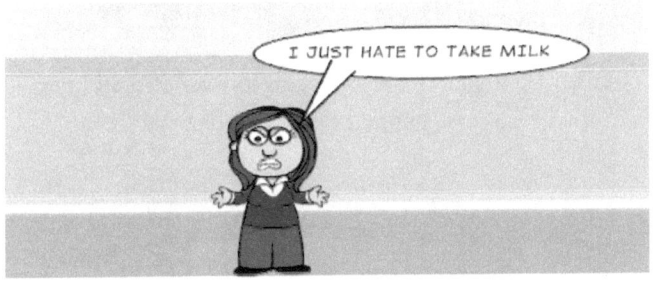

Aversion to milk (Physical Generals - Normal disposition)

Symptoms of altered disposition are those which are observed in the person as a response to the flow of disturbance from the centre to the periphery. These symptoms are not a part of the individual when the person is healthy but is manifested only when the state of health is altered i.e., after the vital force has been deranged. Such symptoms of changed disposition hold atmost value if its very peculiar rare and specific as they reflect the symptoms of early derangement and is a reliable guide in the hunt to reach at the perfect similimum. Here are some examples

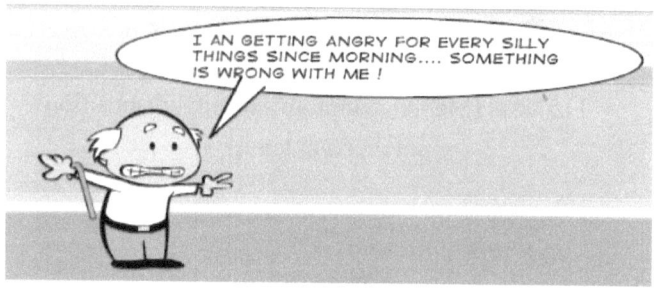

(Anger (Unusual) - Mental symptom emotional level - Changed Disposition)

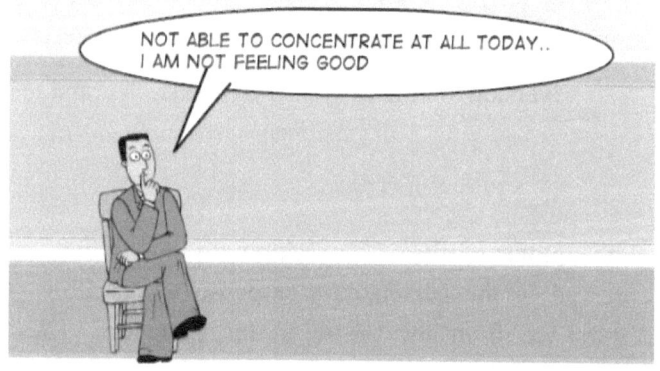

Lack of concentration (Mental symptom - Intellectual level- changed disposition)

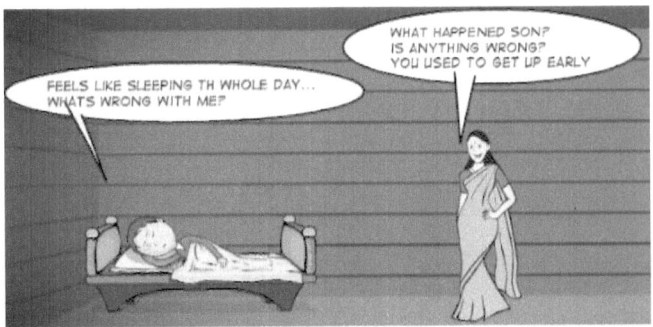

Sleepiness (Physical general - Altered Disposition)

Evaluation of symptoms

Once the case taking is done each and every observed symptom has to be classified as discussed above which shall then help to give the observed symptom a value. This process of giving value to an observed symptom is called as "evaluation of symptoms". It's the value of a given symptom that shall decide whether it shall fit into the totality or not.

FLOW CHART OF SYMPTOM CLASSIFICATION

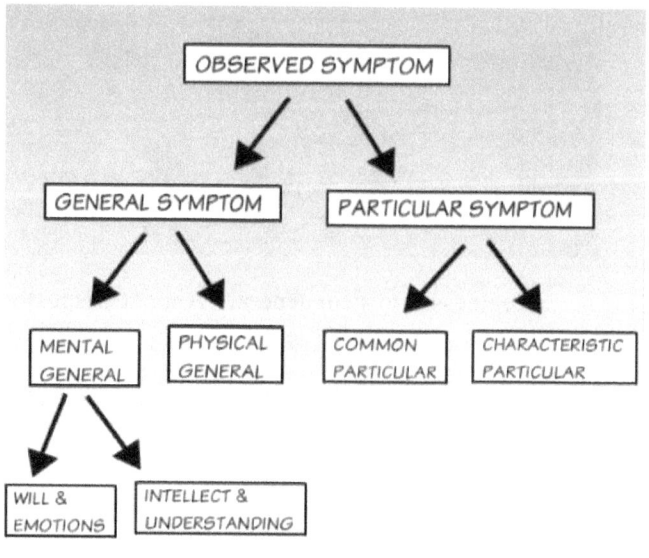

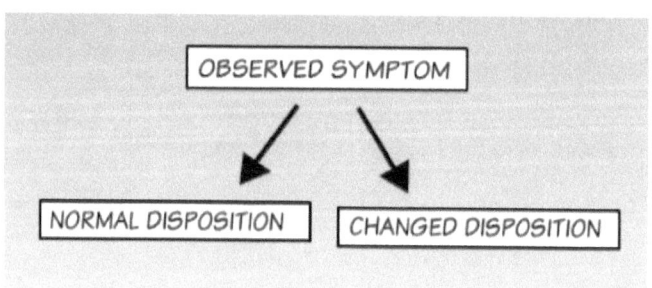

According to their peculiarly and how strange and uncommon they are the symptoms are given value as per the below hierarchy

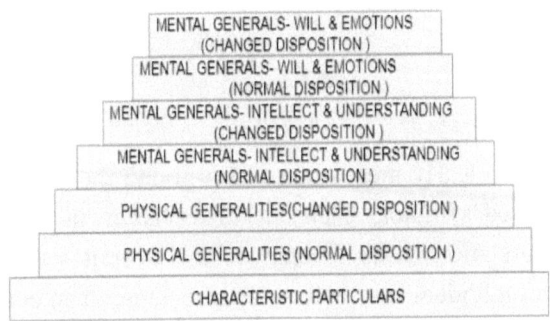

It has to be remembered that the above hierarchy cannot be considered as a rule but its only an indication as to how the observed symptoms has to be given value. The more peculiar, strange and rare a symptom is the more value it deserves to get.

A few strong mental generals can rule out any number of particulars and such strong generals always deserve more weightage while constructing the totality.

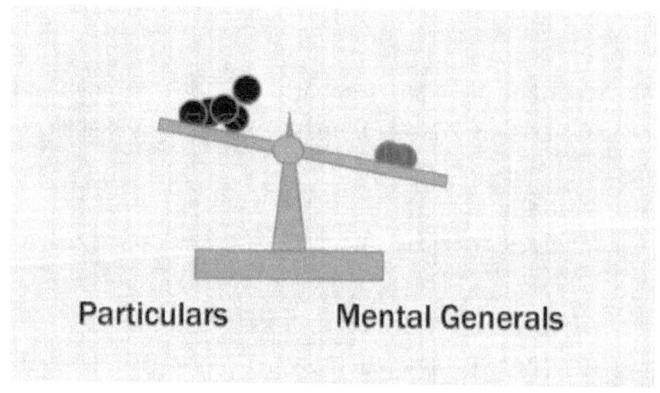

Particulars   **Mental Generals**

This clearly means that while giving the value to an observed symptom each one of us has to use our own interpretation skills to analyze the overall scenario in each individual case before we give value to an observed symptom.

It is equally important for us to have the knowledge of human nature, the normal feelings and reactions in various situations and also to understand the mindset of an individual so that anything observed contrary to what is expected can be easily figured out and such observations deserves to get more weightage while constructing the totality.

6. Case Analysis and Evaluation

Giving value to an observed symptom

Giving value to an observed symptom is a very crucial step that has to be performed with extreme caution and care. If we make a mistake in giving proper value to an observed symptom either that symptoms will get omitted from being included in the totality or unimportant symptoms shall be a part of the totality. In either scenario we may miss out the perfect similimum. So, it becomes very important for us to understand on what basis we give value to an observed symptom.

As a general rule it has to be kept in mind that when we observe something that is not expected to be present it has got high value. Have a look at the example given below

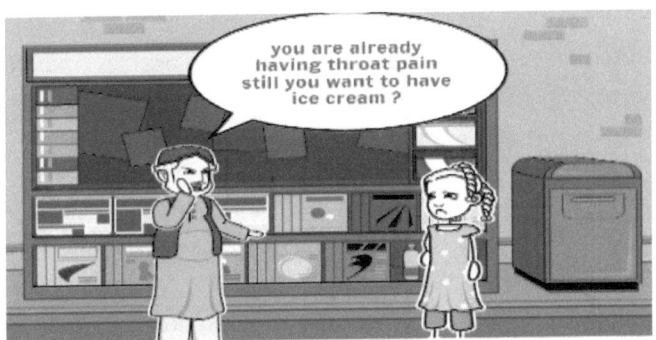

In the above example when someone is having tonsilitis we expect that there shall be an aggravation from taking cold but in a case if you observe that a patient having tonsillitis still has a desire for cold food or drinks then that becomes a symptom which is totally unexpected. Hence such symptoms have high value.

On the other hand, if we expected a symptom to be present but it is not found then that also has a very high value. Look at the example below

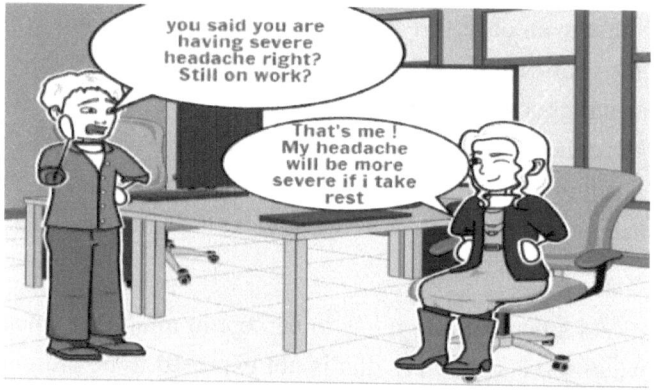

A person having severe headache we expect that complaints to become worse while working (mental strain) so that becomes an expected symptom but when you do not observe it then it has got high value.

So, in a case when you find something that is expected it has less value whereas when you find something that is not expected it has got high value. Similarly, when you do not find something that is expected to be present then it also has got a high value.

Secondly, any observed symptoms that looks strange, rare and peculiar to that individual person it always has a high value. Have a look at the example given below

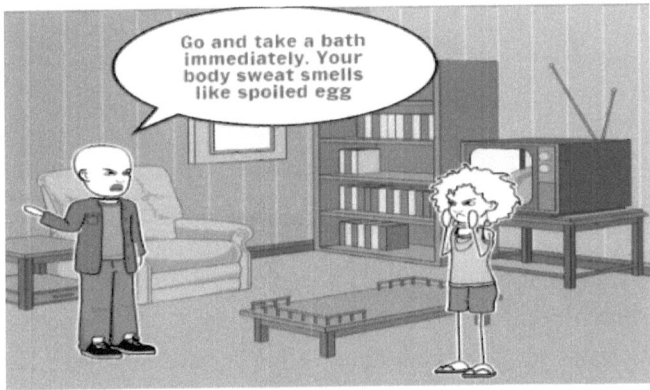

Perspiration smells like rotten egg is a very strange, rare and peculiar symptoms (Physical general in this case) hence it has got high value.

We had already discussed about the symptoms of normal disposition and changed disposition. All those symptoms that belongs to the changed disposition of the patient usually have high value unless they do not become common to the disease thereby losing its value. Consider the example below:

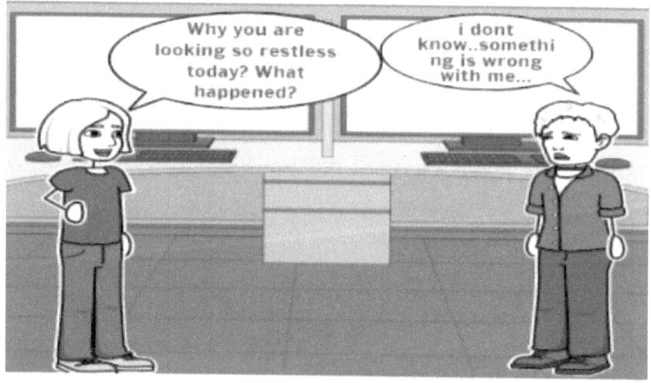

Unusual restlessness is a mental symptom of changed disposition and these symptoms have high value as those belongs to the person and not his disease. On the other hand, consider the example given below.

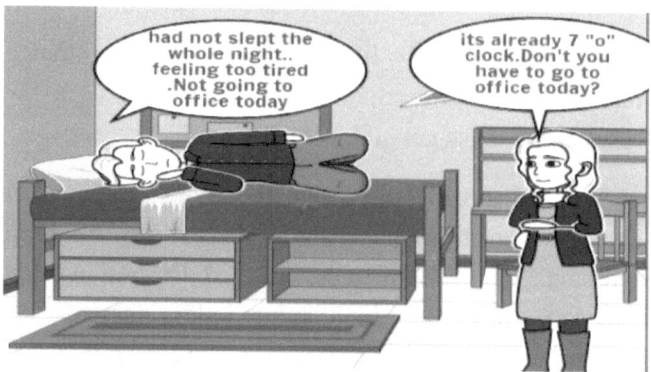

Now here although laziness and tired feeling in the morning are symptoms of changed disposition here the person could not sleep the whole night so tiredness and laziness in the early morning to get up is quite expected and hence it does not have much value.

In short each and every symptom has to be analyzed with proper skill and correct interpretation to be able to judge as to what value does it deserve to get and will that symptom qualify to be considered to form the totality.

There is one more interesting fact to keep in mind that the value of the same symptom varies from person to person and also in the same person in different situations. This means that we cannot award a pre decided value to an observed symptom.

Let's try to understand this with the help of an example.

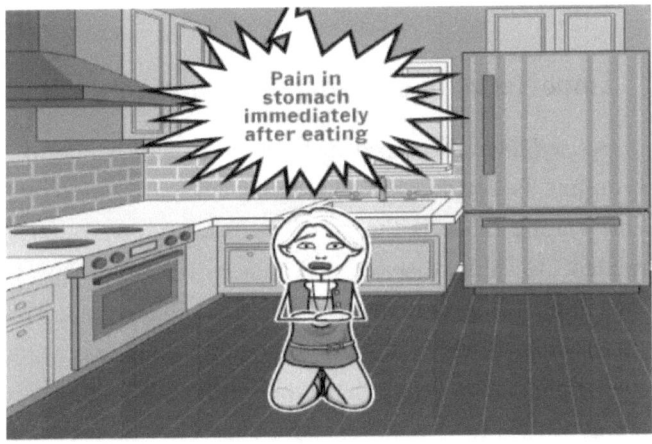

Consider the above symptom pain in stomach immediately after eating. This symptom can be a characteristic particular in a person who let's say is having a migraine. But for someone who is diagnosed with gastric ulcer this same symptom then loses its value and becomes a common symptom as we know that intake of food irritates the damaged gastric mucosa thereby patients having gastric ulcers usually has an aggravation immediately after taking the food.

So, it has to be kept in mind that the same symptom may have different values in two different individuals and also the value may vary in the same individual under different circumstances. Hence before giving value to an observed symptom proper interpretation of the observed symptom becomes very essential and plays an important role in deciding wheather the symptom shall qualify to fit into the final totality of the given case.

Importance of studying allied subjects

As we have discussed just above that the value of a symptom is decided by considering various parameters. One among those is the more an observed symptom is related to the disease (ultimate) or common to the clinical diagnosis made the lesser value it has. This means that all those disease symptoms have less value for helping us to select the right similimum unless they are accompanied by any specific characteristic modality or concomitant. So, in order to list out the uncommon symptoms we should first have a thorough knowledge of the common symptoms related to that particular disease. So, it becomes very essential for us to study these common symptoms on the basis of which such clinical diagnosis is made so that we can easily eliminate them while analyzing the case.

It's also equally important for us to have a good knowledge of anatomy, physiology and pathology. These subjects teach us how a normal body is made up of (anatomy), how it carries out various functioning in a harmonious way (Physiology) and how it reacts and responds to invasions or any factor threatening to cause disharmony (Pathology). This shall help us to identify the symptoms related to the normal defense and self protection process of the body.

Let's consider an example to understand this in a better way.

We all know that inflammation is the body's response towards infection. The five cardinal signs of inflammation include

a) Pain

b) Swelling

c) Redness

d) Heat

e) Loss of function

So when we have any inflammatory condition in hand like bronchitis, tonsillitis or arthritis all the above mentioned symptoms that is pain, swelling, redness, heat and loss of function becomes something we expect to see in the case. Hence these have very less value. But at the same time in such conditions if we observe any expected symptoms to be absent then it shall have very high value. Have a look at the examples given below:

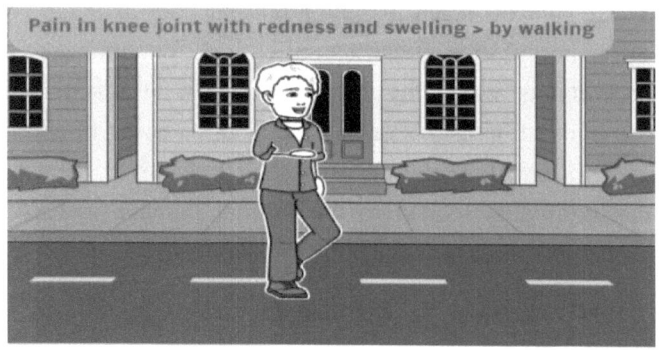

Pain in knee joint with redness and sweling > by walking

In the above example someone who is having pain, swelling and redness (signs of inflammation) in his knee joint we expect his pain to become severe while walking (Loss of function). But in such a case if the patient feels better by walking (Motion) then it is something that is not expected hence will become very important and shall have a very high value in the given case.

To understand this in a better way, let's consider a simple example. Have a look at the image shown below.

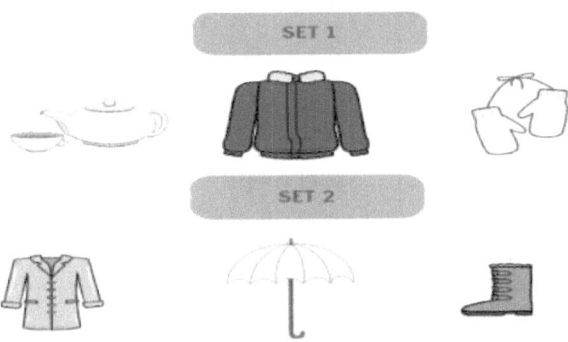

You can see the above two sets of images. The images in SET 1 are those objects which are very useful in winters and cold climates and has least importance in rainy weather. The images in SET 2 are of utmost importance in rainy weather and have least importance in winters and cold climates except tea. So, a hot tea has equal importance in both these climates.

These set of images can be compared with the observed symptoms of a case. Its importance or value is decided by taking into consideration various scenarios.

To summarize the value of a symptom is depended on and is decided by various parameters which include:

a. How uncommon, strange and peculiar they are in the given case.

b. When it is accompanied by a very specific modality or concomitant

c. When it is unexpected to be found but present.

d. When it is expected to be present but absent.

e. When it is specific to the individual person and not common to his disease suffering.

Importance of clinical diagnosis in Homoeopathy

In the earlier sections we had discussed that a clinical diagnosis is made taking into consideration those set of common symptoms which are observed commonly in all or majority of people having the same disease. It can also be said that clinical diagnosis is a name given to the "disease ultimates".

We had already discussed that homoeopathic remedy for a given case is not selected on the basis of disease ultimates but those individualistic symptoms belonging to the patient both at mental and physical level has to be grouped together to form the totality and it is this totality that decides the remedy. So, it becomes very evident from this discussion that it is not important for us to make a precise clinical diagnosis for selecting the homeopathic remedy. As Dr Kent has said "Except in a few acute diseases no diagnosis can be made, and no diagnosis need be made except that the patient is sick. The more one thinks of the name of a disease so called the more one is beclouded in the search for a remedy, for then the mind is only upon the result of the disease, and not upon the image expressed in symptoms."

Here it is emphasised again that we need to look for the image of sickness through the symptoms expressed and that image has to matched exactly with the image reflected by a remedy which then shall fit in as the perfect similimum for the given case.

To understand this more clearly, let's consider the totality of a person having bronchial asthma. (See below: Refer Kent's Repertory)

Mind, anguish, driving from place to place (p. 3)

Mind, anxiety, alone, when (p. 5)

Mind, censorious, critical (p. 10)

Stomach, desires, cold drinks (p. 484)

Stomach, thirst, small quantities, for (p. 529)

Respiration, asthmatic, night, midnight, after (p. 764)

Respiration, difficult, cough, with (p. 768)

Respiration, difficult, turning in bed (p. 772)

As per the above totality if we repertorize the case then Arsenicum Album shall cover all the above symptoms in first grade thereby fitting in as the perfect similimum for this given case of a patient having bronchial asthma. Now, let's imagine that the same patient is having migraine instead of bronchial asthma and let's construct the totality accordingly.

Mind, anguish, driving from place to place (p. 3)

Mind, anxiety, alone, when (p. 5)

Mind, censorious, critical (p. 10)

Stomach, desires, cold drinks (p. 484)

Stomach, thirst, small quantities, for (p. 529)

Head, pain, forehead, eyes, above, warm applications amel. (p. 161)

Head, pain, burning, forehead, eyes, over, night (p. 177)

Head, pain, walking in open air, amel. (p. 151)

As you can see if the above totality is repertorized still Arsenicum Album would be the remedy. So, it becomes very evident that as long as the quality symptoms of patient fits in with the remedy it shall remain unchanged irrespective of the disease ultimate that the patient is diagnosed with. So clinical diagnosis doesn't hold much importance in selecting a homoeopathic remedy.

Sometimes we see many patient's roaming in and out of various speciality clinics consulting the so called specialists to get rid of their complaints. But, when the changes are observed only at general level and nothing can be found on the outermost physical plane nor anything abnormal can be traced through the microscopes or laboratory investigation the modern school prefer to wait until to observe some changes at physical level so that they could give a name to the observed changes. They usually cannot begin their treatment unless the disease has not been given a diagnostic name. They even restrain to call the person as sick despite having abnormality at general level in the form of abnormal sensations or functioning and shall declare the person to have "no disease".

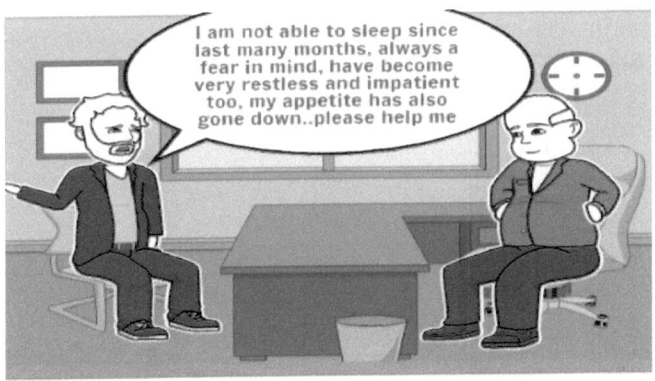

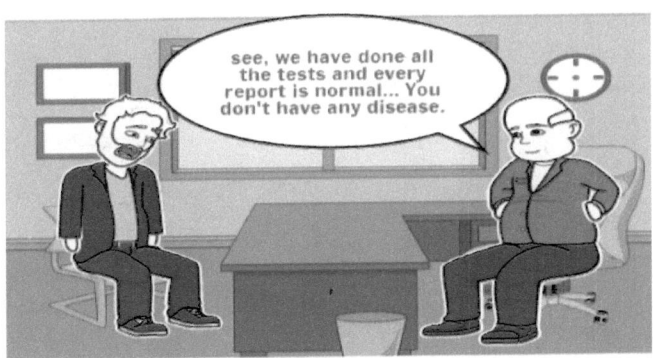

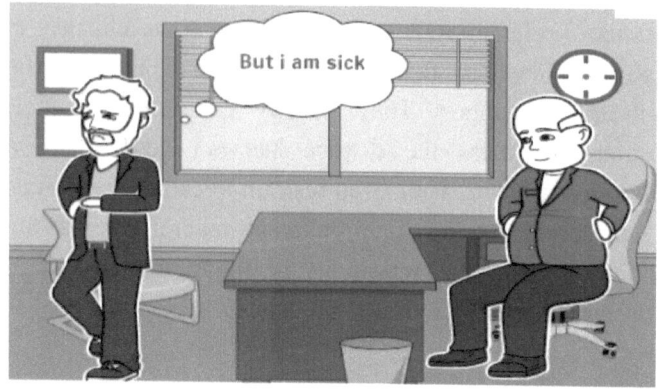

In such cases they prefer to wait until they can trace something at physical level and in many cases by that time the disease would have progressed to such an extent to render the case as incurable.

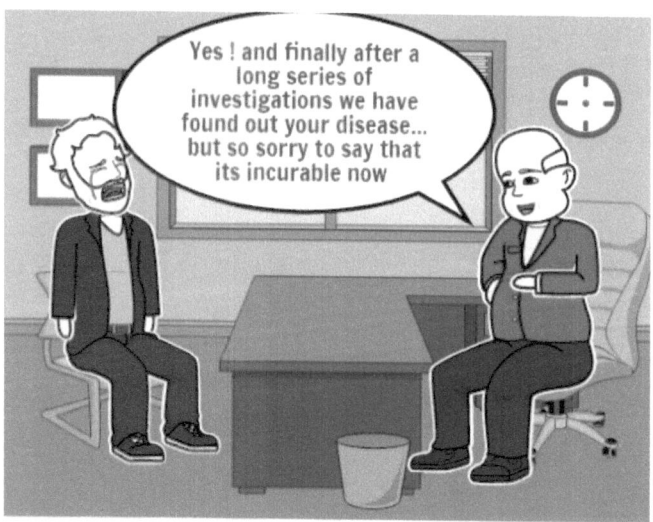

It is the patient who becomes sick and not his individual parts or organs, so it is the patient who has to be treated not his individual part or organ. Let's quote the reference from our literature to understand this more precisely

"Under traditional methods it is necessary that a diagnosis be made before the treatment can be settled, but in most cases the diagnosis cannot be made until the results of disease have rendered the patient incurable. (J T Kent)"

However, this doesn't mean that a homeopath have no need to arrive at the precise clinical diagnosis. Reaching at the correct clinical diagnosis has its own importance. It shall help you to access and judge the curability of a case and accordingly the treatment plan can be decided whether to go for curative or palliative treatment. It shall also help you find out the changes in organs, how far the disease has advanced and whether those advancements could be reversed or not.

"Physical diagnosis is very important in its own place. By means of physical diagnosis the physician may find out the changes in organs, how far the disease has progressed, and determine if the patient is incurable. It is necessary also in supplying information to Boards of Health.It may also decide whether you should give curative or palliative treatments (J T Kent)"

Totality of a case

All observed symptoms in a case are not equally important. In each and every case there are some peculiar strange rare and characteristic symptoms. These set of symptoms when grouped together and rearranged according to their respective values forms the totality of that case.

So, it can be said that the totality of a case are those set of important symptoms in a case that are peculiar, strange and rare. These symptoms hold a crucial value in guiding us towards the right similimum. Totality of a case is the backbone upon which the entire case stands erect. If the totality is not constructed perfectly our case will not stand erect and we shall never be able to reach at the perfect similimum. It has been discussed earlier the importance of giving value to an observed symptom. If one goes wrong in giving proper value to an observed symptom then he shall also fail to construct a perfect totality. The totality thus formed when logically rearranged in order of their value and importance refelects an image know as the image of sickness or portrait of disease.

Repertorial totality

Totality of a case is formed by the important symptoms of a given case arranged logically in order of their importance. These symptoms when converted into the language of repertory in the form of rubrics give rise the "Repertorial totality". So, the difference between the totality of a case and repertorial totality is that in the later the symptoms are in the form of rubrics. For example, if in the totality of a case there is a symptom "desire for company", the same symptom when fits into the repertorial totality becomes "Mind, company, desire for". As it can be seen that in totality of a case the symptom is mentioned in patient's language whereas in repertorial totality it is converted into its appropriate rubric.

Potential Differential Field (PDF)

There can be instances where one may observe a very important symptom in a case that deserves to fit into the case totality but there may not be any specific rubric avialable for the given symptom in the repertory. In such a situation the observed symptom cannot fit in to the repertorial totality. Such group of symptoms which fail to fit into the repertorial totality because of the non-avialability of the specific rubric for that given symptom are grouped together to form the "Potential Differential field".

Importance or utlity of PDF: The final remedy cannot be selected only on the bais of repertorization as it only helps to short list a few important remedies that could be the final similimum. From the repertorial result the remedies that have come up has to again studied and compared to reach at the final similimum. The symptoms listed in the PDF plays a very important role in helping to reach at the right similimum. It has to be cross checked as to which remedy from the repertorial result cover the symptoms is listed in the PDF.

Sometimes there is also a possibility that we may not be sure about the validity of an observed symptom because of lack of clarity and information. In such cases when we are in doubt it is ideally recommended to keep such symptoms in the PDF to be compared at the end for the final selection of the remedy.

Repertorization and Repertorial result

Once the reportorial totality has been constructed the next step is the repertorization. The method of repertorization has been discussed in detail in the following chapter. However, it has to be kept in mind that the selection of repertory and the method of repertorization depends on the final case totality. Also, every repertory is based on a certain philosophical background and depending on that the totality has to be rearranged to get the best results out of repertorization.

Once the rpertorization is done the top three or four remedies obtaining highest marks are listed down in the Oder of the marks obtained. This arrangement forms the reportorial result.

Selecting the final remedy

It has to be kept in mind that the remedy obtaining the highest marks after repertorization need not be the right similimum. The final remedy has to be selected after consulting the symptoms listed in the PDF followed by referring the materia medica and reading all the drugs listed under the reportorial result. So ultimately it is the materia medica that forms the base for the final selection of a remedy. Repertorization is a tool that shall ensure that this laborious task of hunting for the right similimum for a given case is made easy.

7. Boenninghausen's Thereupeutic pocket book

The "Therapeutic Pocket Book" was published in 1846 by Boenninghausen. The orginal name of the book was "Therapeutic Pocket Book for Homoeopathic Physicians to use at the Bedside and in the Study of the Materia Medica". The orginal version included 126 remedies. Allen's edited translation is the one which is mostly in use and popular. He added 220 remedies to the Boenninghausen's original 126 remedies and so in total 342 remedies are included in the Allen's edition.

Philosophic Background

Boenninghausen's "Therapeutic Pocket book" is based on the concept of complete symptom. According to him a symptom is said to be complete when it has the following components:

a) Location

b) Sensation

c) Modalities

d) Concomitant (not mandatory)

So, in order to use the "Therapeutic pocket book" one need to have a complete symptom in hand and practically there were some difficulties in tracing the complete symptom from the patient. So, in oder to complete the symptom he evolved some fundamental concepts on the basis of which this book is based. These are as follows:

1) <u>Doctrine of Analogy</u>: This principle is also called as "Doctrine of Grand Generalization". According to this the local modalities and sensations pertaining to one part should also be applied to other parts. This means he raised the local modalities and sensations to a general level that can then applied to the other parts as well. This helped to make the symptom complete.

2) <u>Doctrine of Concomitants</u>: Concomitant symptoms are those symptoms which appear along with the chief complaints but shall have no physiological or pathological relationship with the chief complaints. The presence of these symptoms cannot be explained logically and appear to very strange, rare and peculiar to the concerned individual. They play an important role in Individualizing the case as well as the remedy.

3) <u>Evaluation of Remedies</u>: The remedies have been listed under five grades in "Theurapeutic pocket book"

a) In CAPITALS carrying 5 marks (Grade 1)

b) In **Bold** carrying 4 marks (Grade 2)

c) In *italics* carrying 3 marks (Grade 3)

d) In Roman carrying 2 marks (Grade 4)

e) In (Roman) within brackets carrying 1 mark. (Grade 5)

This gradation is based on the frequency and intensity of the apperaence of symptoms in provers. That is the remedies listed in first grade are higly reliable whereas the remedies listed in fifth grade are least reliable.

4) Conordances: In this chapter the relationship that exist among the remedies are listed under various headings including antidotes and inicimals.

Plan and construction:

This book begins with the mind and intellect chapter. Further the book has been divided into three parts

a) Location

b) Sensation and

c) Modalities

The mind chapter contains only 18 rubrics wheras the intellect contains only 17 rubrics. Although concomitants are given high importance there is no separate chapter included for concomitants and the same is found scattered under other chapters. Towards the end there is a separate chapter on "Relatioship of remedies".

Clinical utility of BTPB

Boenninghausen's therapeutic pocketbook is still quite useful and popular among many especially at bedside or in acute cases where the remedy needs to be selected in the shortest possible time. This reperoty is useful in cases

1) Where there is lack of generals

2) Where there are prominent sensations and modalities

3) Where the symptom is complete

Method of working out a case

A) Robert's Method

After the completion of case taking the observed symptoms are rearranged under the following heads:

1. Location
2. Sensations
3. Modalities
4. Concomitants

Post repertorization the mental symptoms are used for differentiation and final selection of remedy.

B) Modern Method

According to this method after the case taking, the symptoms are rearranged in the following hierarchy

1. Causitive modalities (Emotional, Intellectual and physical)
2. General aggravations (Emotional, Intellectual and physical)
3. General ameliorations (Emotional, Intellectual and physical)
4. Physical generals: Sensation and complaints
5. Concomitants

Mentals for reference and differentiation

8. Boger Boenninghausen's Characteristics and Repertory (B.B.C.R)

With the ever growing list of remedies it was becoming very difficult for the practitioners to find out the correct similimum in the shortest possible time. Theurapeutic pocket was although of great use till then it also had some drawbacks and disadvantages.

To overcome the drawbacks and criticisms of theurapeutic pocket book Boger undertook the work of rewriting the Boenninghausen's repertory. He added aggravations, ameliorations and concomitants in a detail at the end of every chapter. He included 464 medicines in his reperory. It also contains characteristics of medicines in the first part and the repertory in the second part. Hence the book is given the name Boenninghausen's characteristics and repertory.

Philosophical background

B.B.C.R is based on the following basic fundamental concepts:

1) Doctirne of complete symptoms and concomitants

2) Doctrine of pathological generals

3) Doctrine of causation and time

4) Clinical rubrics

5) Evaluation of remedies

6) Fever totality

7) Concordances

Doctrine of complete symptoms and concomitants:

Boger also adopted the concept of complete symptom as given by Boenninghausen. A complete symptom is one which consists of location, sensations and modalities. Concomitants may or may not present. The concept of constructing the totality is same as given by Boenninghausen but he further added sensation and modalities to specific parts. Concomitants are given at most importance and is listed in realtion to the parts.

Doctrine of pathological generals:

When the same pathological changes are observed at more than one part or in general realted to the person as a whole they become pathological generals. They are of great importance in constructing the totality. Example Atrophy, discharges, dropsy, swellings, inflammations etc.

Doctrine of causation and time:

Boger in his work has given great importance to the causation and time of expressions. At the end of each chapter time aggravation has been given which also contains many causative factors. When found well marked in a case, the causative factors and characteristic modalities play a key role in forming the totality of the given case.

Clinical Rubrics:

In some cases where there is a lack of quality individualistic and characteristic symptoms these clinical rubrics may be used to select the remedy. However, this method is not advocated and should be put to a limited use as the disease ultimates do not decide the remedy. In acute conditions to bring down the intensity of symptoms when characteristic symptoms are lacking thiese clinical rubrics are useful.

Evaluation of remedies

Boger followed the same type of gradings which Boenninghausen followed.

a) CAPITAL – 5 Marks

b) **Bold** - 4 Marks

c) *Italics* - 3 Marks

d) Roman - 2 Marks

e) (Roman) – 1 Mark

The gradation is based on the frequency of appearance of symptoms in prvers.

Fever Totality

In this chapter the rubrics are arranged in a simple and easy way to use clinically. The three stages of fever ie the chill, heat and perspiration is followed by the time aggravation, amelioration and concomitant.

Concordances:

This chapter deals with the relationship of remedies. It covers 125 remedies.

Plan and construction

The book contains in total 53 chapters as given below

1) Mind

2) Sensorium

3) Vertigo

4) Head

5) Eyes

6) Ears

7) Nose

8) Face

9) Teeth

10) Mouth

11) Appetite

12) Thirst

13) Tatse

14) Eructation

15) Waterbrash and Heartburn

16) Hiccough

17) Nausea and Vomiting

18) Stomach

19) Epigastrium

20) Hypochondria

21) Abdomen

22) External Abdomen

23) Inguinal and Pubic region

24) Flatulance

25) Stool

26) Aus and rectum
27) Perineum
28) Prostate gland
29) Urine
30) Urinary organs
31) Gentalia – (Male organs, Female organs)
32) Sexual Impulse
33) Menstruation
34) Respiration
35) Cough
36) Larynx and Trachea
37) Voice and speech
38) Neck and external throat
39) Chest
40) Back
41) Upper extremities
42) Lower extremities
43) Sensations and complaints in general
44) Glands
45) Bones
46) Skin and exterior body

47) Sleep

48) Dreams

49) Fever

50) Compound fevers

51) Conditions in general

52) Conditions of aggravations and ameliorations in general

53) Concordances

The rubrics are arranged in each chapter under the headings of location and sensations (mixed) followed by time modalities of aggravations and ameliorations. In some chapters concomitants are listed separately.

Methods of Repertorization

There are several ways to work out a case using BBCR depending upon what we have in the given case.

1) <u>Using Causitive modalities</u>: When the caistive factor or modalities are known those can be considered at first place and form the totality in the given below hierarchy:

-Causitive modalities (Including ailments from)

- Other modalities –

    Aggravations (Mental and physical)

Ameliorations (Mental and Physical)

- Physical generals

- Concomitants

- Location and sensations

2) <u>Using modalities</u>: In cases where we do not have causitive modalities but only general or particular modalities the case can be repertorized by constructing the totality in below order:

- Modalities – (mental and Physical)

- Concomitants

- Physical Generals

- Location and sensations

3) <u>Using concomitants</u>: In cases where we have well defined strong concomitant symptoms the case can be repertorized by forming the totality in the below order:

- Concomitants

-Modalities

-Physical Genrals

- Location and sensations

4) <u>Using Pathological Genrals</u>: In cases having pathological generals the totality can be formed as given below:

- Pathological Generals
- Physical Generals
- Concomitants
- Modalities

5) <u>Using Diagnostic or clinical rubrics</u>: Diagnostic or clinical rubrics should ideally be put into limited use and only in those cases where we do not have any other quality symptom to work with. The totality can be formed as given below

- Clinical Rubric
- Aggravations
- Ameliorations
- Weak concomitants
- Physical generals

6) <u>Following Theurapeutic pocket book method</u>

- Locations and sensations
- Modalities
- Concomitants
- Physical generals

7) <u>Fever totality</u>: In handling cases of fever this chapter is quite convenient to use. Symptoms of chill stage, heat stage and sweat stage are listed down in the order of their type, time, aggravation, amelioration and concomitant.

9. Kent's Repertory

Introduction

Reperory of the homoeopathic materia medica by J T Kent is still the most popular repertory in use even today. It was published in the year 1897. Kent emphasized on giving importance to the person as a whole. His holistic approach and his explanations on the basic principles of Homeopathy gives a clarity and guidance to the practitioners. The number of medicines used in this repertory is 648.

Philosophic background

Kent's repertory is based on the philosophy of deductive logic i.e., from generals to particulars. Our body is made up two planes

a) Materialistic plane

b) Dynamic plane

The outermost materialistic plane is composed of all the cells tissues, organs, nerves and blood vessels. The inner most dynamic plane is composed of the vital force as the central controlling unit, our will and emotions and intellect and understanding.

Vital force once deranged creates an imbalance which flows from the centre to the periphery affecting first will & emotions then intellect & understanding, then the physical generalities are altered and finally the physical symptoms appear. So, in accordance with this flow of disturbance the observed symptoms are given priority in oder of its appearance as given below:

1) Mental symptoms: Will and emotional level

2) Mental symptoms: Intellect and understanding level

3) Physical generalities

4) Characteristic particulars

Grading of remedies

In kent's repertory the remedies are listed under three grades.

First garde symptoms are those which are indicated in Bold letter. They are those symptoms which are felt strongly by all the provers or majority of provers. They are highly reliable and carry 3 marks.

Second grade symptoms are those which have been brought out by few provers which are not confirmed but occasionally verified. They carry 2 marks.

Third grade symptoms are those which are brought out by prvers now and then and are not confirmed by reproving. They are least relaible and carry 1 mark each.

Kent's concept of totality

Kent classified the symptoms into general and paricular. General symptoms are further divided into mental generals and physical generals.

Mental generals include symptoms related to

1) <u>Will & Emotions</u>: Like anger, sadness, depression, love, hatred, fear, grief, anxiety etc.

2) <u>Intellect and Understanding</u>: Like absent-minded, delusions, illusions, hallucinations, speech, memory, understanding etc

Physical generals include symptoms related to

a. Appetite

b. Desires & Avesrions

c. Thirst

d. Prespiration

e. Sleep

f. Menstruation

g. Urination

h. Bowel habits

i. Symptoms related to sexual sphere

j. General aggaravations & Amelorations

k. Weather impacts

Particular symptoms are further divided into two categories

1) Common particulars

2) Characteristic particulars

While constructing the totality mental symptoms realted to will and emotions are given high priority followed by mental symptoms realted to intellect and understanding. Then physical generalities are considered (based on their pecularity) and finally characteristic particulars are taken into account. So, it becomes very clear that Kent has given least importance to the symptoms common to the disease.

A totality thus constructed in an oderly way shall cover the symptoms of the patient as a whole and the remedy selected on the basis of such a totality shall fit in perfectly with the peculairities of the patient.

Plan and construction

Kent has given prime importance to the mental symptoms. Hence kent's repertory starts with the mind chapter and followed by chapters listed in anatomical divisions followed by function or discharges. These chapters include

1) Mind

2) Vertigo

3) Head

4) Eye

5) Vision

6) Ear

7) Hearing

8) Nose

9) Face

10) Mouth

11) Teeth

12) Throat

13) External throat

14) Stomach

15) Abdomen

16) Rectum

17) Stool

18) Urinary organs

a) Bladder

b) Kidney

c) Proststate gland

d) Urethra

e) Urine

19) Genitalia – Male

20) Genitalia – Female
21) Larynx and Trachea
22) Respiration
23) Cough
24) Expectoration
25) Chest
26) Back
27) Extremities
28) Sleep
29) Chill
30) Fever
31) Prespiration
32) Skin
33) Generalities

Arrangement of rubrics

In Kent's repertory a rubric starts with a general symptom or state listed in capital bold with a list of remedies listed against it. This is called as the main rubric.

±± **ABANDONED** (See Forsaken)

±± **ABRUPT** : Nat-m., *tarent.*

±± **ABSENT-MINDED** (See Forgetful) : *Acon.*, act-sp., æsc., agar., *agn.*, all-c., *alum., am-c.,* am-m., *anac.,* ang., **Apis.**, arg-m., *arn.,* ars., arum-t., asar., *aur., bar-c.,* **bell., bov.,** *bufo-r., calad.,* calc-s., calc., **Cann-i.,** cann-s., caps., carb-ac., carb-s., *carl.,* **Caust.,** cench., **Cham.,** chel., chin., *cic.,* clem., *cocc.,* coff., *colch.,* coloc., con., croc., crot-h., *cupr.,* cycl., daph., dirc., dulc., elaps., *graph.,* guai., ham., **Hell.,** hep., hura., *hyos., ign.,* jug-c., *kali-br., kali-c., kali-p.,* kali-s., *kreos., lac-c.,* **Lach.,** led., *lyc.,* lyss., *mag-c.,* manc., mang., *merc.,* **Mez.,** *mosch.,* naja., nat-c., **Nat-m.,** nat-p., nit-ac., **Nux-m.,** *nux-v., ohnd., onos., op., petr., ph-ac., phos.,* **Plat.,** *plb.,* **Puls.,** rhod., *rhus-t.,* rhus-v., ruta., sars., **Sep.,** *sil.,* spong., stann., stram., sul-ac., *sulph.,* tarent., thu., **Verat.,** verb., viol-o., viol-t., zinc.

In the above image the rubrics ABANDONED, ABRUPT and ABSENT MINDED listed in **CAPITAL BOLD** are called as the "main rubric". It can also be seen that against the first main rubric ABANDONED no remedies are listed but instead in brackets it is mentioned as (See forsaken). This rubric mentioned within brackets is known as the "cross reference"

Against the main rubric ABSENT-MINDED remedies are listed in three grades. The remedies listed in **bold** are the first grade symptoms. Those listed in *italics* are the second grade symptoms whereas those listed in normal font are the thrid grade symptoms.

±± **ABSENT-MINDED** (See Forgetful) : *Acon.*, act-sp., æsc., agar., *agn.*, all-c., *alum., am-c.,* am-m., *anac.,* ang., **Apis.**, arg-m., *arn.,* ars., arum-t., asar., *aur., bar-c.,* **bell., bov.,** *bufo-r., calad.,* calc-s., calc., **Cann-i.,** cann-s., caps., carb-ac., carb-s., *carl.,* **Caust.,** cench., **Cham.,** chel., chin., *cic.,* clem., *cocc.,* coff., *colch.,* coloc., con., croc., crot-h., *cupr.,* cycl., daph., dirc., dulc., elaps., *graph.,* guai., ham., **Hell.,** hep., hura., *hyos., ign.,* jug-c., *kali-br., kali-c., kali-p.,* kali-s., *kreos., lac-c.,* **Lach.,** led., *lyc.,* lyss., *mag-c.,* manc., mang., *merc.,* **Mez.,** *mosch.,* naja., nat-c., **Nat-m.,** nat-p., nit-ac., **Nux-m.,** *nux-v., ohnd., onos., op., petr., ph-ac., phos.,* **Plat.,** *plb.,* **Puls.,** rhod., *rhus-t.,* rhus-v., ruta., sars., **Sep.,** *sil.,* spong., stann., stram., sul-ac., *sulph.,* tarent., thu., **Verat.,** verb., viol-o., viol-t., zinc.

±± morning : Guai., nat-c., ph-ac., phos.

±± 11 a.m. to 4 p.m. : Kali-n.

±± noon : Mosch.

±± menses, during : Calc.

±± periodical attacks of, short lasting : Fl-ac., *nux-m.*

±± reading, while : Agn., lach., *nux-m.,* ph-ac.

±± starts when spoken to : Carb-ac.

In the above image under the main rubric ABSENT MINDED some more rubrics are listed as subheadings under the main rubric like morning, menses during etc. These are called as the sub rubrics. A main general rubric containing a vast number of remedies listed against it, usually becomes a vague rubric and have least value unless it is not very strage and peculiar to the given case.

Sub rubrics that have only a handful of remedies listed against it also have a limited importance while repertorizing a case unless it is very strage rare and peculiar symptom of the given case. Such rubrics are often used to differentiate the final few remedies from the repertorial result.

Method of working out a case

There are two methods to work out a case using Kent's repertory.

a) Addition method

b) Eliminating method

Addition method

In addition methods once the totality of the case has been constructed the repertorization is done taking into equal account all the rurbics from the repertorial totality.

For example, let's consider the repertorial totality of a case as given below:

1) Fear, alone of being
2) Comapany, desire for
3) Mind, absent minded
4) Mind, speech, confused
5) Vertigo, rising on agg
6) Stomach, desire sweets
7) Respiration difficult, walking rapildy (agg)
8) Respiration, dificult, air, in cold amel

In repertorization using addition method all rubrics are given equal importance the repertorial result would be

Puls 14/6

Phos 14/5

Kali carb 13/6

Eliminating method

In eliminating method one or two most important symptoms of the given case are considered as the eliminating symptom(s) and for the remaining rubrics in the repertorial totality only those remedies are considered which covers either one or both of the eliminating symptoms.

This method has some advantages. It ensures that the final selected remedy covers the most important symptoms of the given case. This method is time saving and goes easy to short list remedies for final selection.

So, an eliminating symptom is the most important symptoms of a given case without considering which the final remedy cannot be slected. They act as filters to rule out other unimportant remedies.

However, it has to be kept in mind that while selecting the eliminating symptom for a given case some precautions has to be considered as follows:

1) The symptom considered should be the most important one from the given case without considering which a similimum cannot be thought of getting selected.

2) It should preferably be a general symptom ideally a mental general which is very starnge rare and peculiar for the given case.

3) The symptom should be well defined and should not be a very vague one having plenty of remedies listed against its corresponding rubric in the repertory. For example, rubrics like irritable, anger, confusion all these are vague rubrics having plenty of remedies listed against it. Such rubrics should be avoided from being considered as an eliminating symptom.

4) Those symptoms which have a very few remedies listed against its corresponding rubric should also be avoided from being considered as an eliminating symptom.

5) In acute cases the causative factor can ideally be considered as an eliminating symptom provided the case does not have any other strong characteristic mental symptoms to gain more weightage.

6) Disease symptoms should not be taking into account for being considered as an eliminating symptom.

It has to be kept in mind that if the eliminating symptoms are not wisely selected then the chances are there that the right similimum shall get ruled out and one may end up selecting a partial similimum.

10. General Topics

Limitations of Homoeopathy

Homoeopathy indeed has got several advanatges over other system of medicines. However, at the same time it also has to be kept in mind that in Homoeopathy there are certain limitations as well. It is very important for us to keep in mind these limitations as well. These limitations include

1) Cases with advanced irreversible changes: In cases where there has been an irreversible damage done homoeopathy has its limitations. For example, we all know that brain cells cannot regenerate. So, in cases where there has been a damage to brain cells it becomes incurable. Also, at the same time patients who have their one or more organs surgically removed there is also a limitation to completely cure the person.

2) Emergency cases which can be fatal: Our remedies act upon the vital force and stimulate it which then removes the disease thereby curing the person. In emergency cases which can be fatal like snake bites or cardiac arrest where there is not enough time for the vitality to react our rmedies has its limitations. In such cases if no proper medical attention is given there are chances that the patient may die. Hence our remedies have very limited role to play in such conditions. However even in such emergency conditions our

remedies can be given to handle the situation until the patient gets a proper aid. In such cases the remedy and potency have to be slected very wisely. To handle such emergency conditions a good clinical experience comes in handy.

3) In cases of severe accidents: In accident cases the vitality is disturbed but not deranged. In such cases there is no true diease to be removed and hence our remedies have limted role to play in such situations. In accidents the injury or damage is limited to the materialistic plane and as we had discussed the dynamic and materialistic planes cannot exist in isolation.

4) In some surgical cases: Homoeopathy can definitely help to avoid surgery in many cases by curing the patient with our remedies like in cases of renal calculi, uterine fibroid or tumours. However, in some advanced cases surgery cannot be avoided and our remedies have a limited role to play in such cases. For example, third degree prolapses.

Advantages of Homeopathy

Homoeopathy has got several advantages over the conventional system of medicine. These are as follows:

1) Rapid and gentle cure: Usually it is believed that homeopathic remedies are slow in acting. However, the fact is that Homoeopathic remedies acts much faster than the allopathic medicines. In acute cases Homoeopathy has the potential to "Abort" the progress of an acute

disease which no other system can do. (discussed previously, Chapter-Case taking: Managing acute cases)

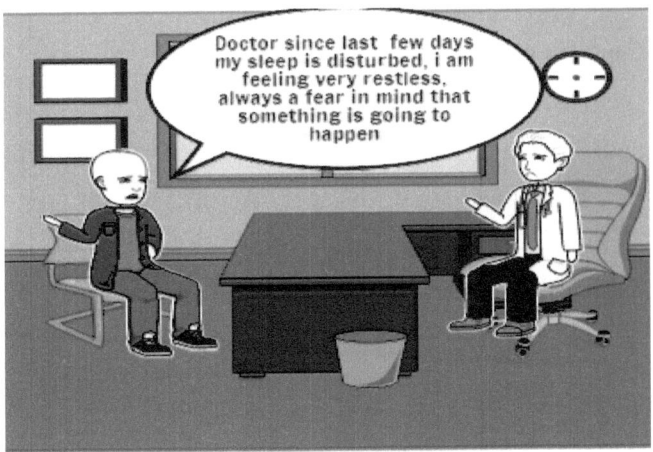

In cases as shown above, a homeopath can prescribe a remedy based only on the initial changes to "Abort" the diease and prevent the appearance of physical symptoms.

2) Complete and permanent cure: Homeopathy is well known for uprooting the chronic cases and curing the patient permenantely. This potential gives our system an upper hand as others only tend to palliate or remove the physical symptoms temporarily.

3) Boost the immunity: Well selected homoeopathic remedies shall boost the general immunity of an individual thereby preventing one from falling sick even after getting exposed to exciting factors that may trigger a disease.

4) Prevention in Epidemics: A well selected remedy (Genus epidemicus) during an epidemic attack shall help to serve as a preventive medicine protecting the mass population from falling sick.

5) In surgical cases: Homoeopathy can help to avoid unnecessary surgeries in cases like uterine fibroids, tumors, caluli etc.

6) Role in incurable cases: Homoeopathy has produced miraculous results even in those cases considered as incurable like cancers.

Obstacles to cure

Sometimes even well selected remedy may fail to yield the expected result. This can happen if there are some obstacles to cure. Some of these obstacles can be removed while a few others cannot be removed. In cases where these obstacles cannot be removed shall render that case incurable and palliation becomes the only option. Some of the factors that act an as obstacle are:

1) Miasms: In some cases, misams may act as an obstacle. It has been discussed earlier (Chapter No. 3) that miasms account for the individual reactions to a stimulus and individual feelings or emotions including the will power. Our remedies however well selected it may be cannot act against the will of an individual. If the patient does not want to get his disease removed or has lost all hope of any possible recovery this may act as a obstacle to cure. In such cases a detailed case taking and

giving proper attention, care, consolation, motivation and support to the patient may help to remove these obstacles. If the patient is in negative frame of mind that shall also sometimes act as an obstacle and in such cases the well selected remedy may not yield the expected result. One such example wherein the patient himself does not wish to get cured is given below:

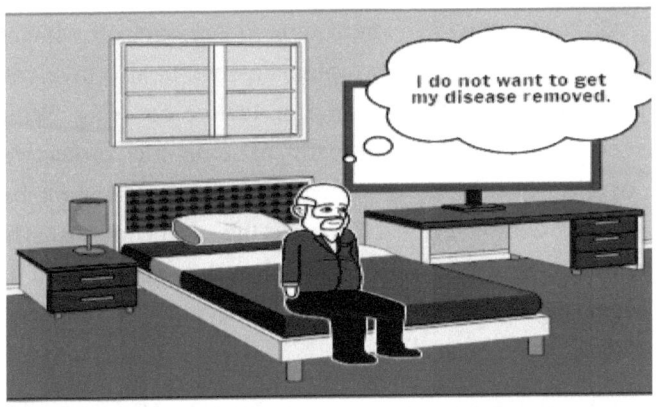

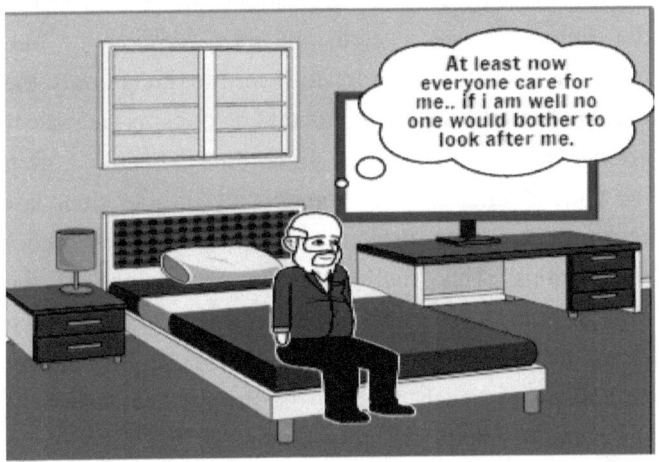

2) Maintaining cause: Presence of maintaining cause can also act as an obstacle to cure. In cases where this maintaining cause can be removed the cure shall follow. But in those cases where it is not posible to remove the maintaining cause the case shall remain incurable and one may not get the expected result from a well selected remedy.

3) Age factor: Complete cure does not only mean removing the physical symptoms alone but also involves in strengthening the dynamic protective covering. With ageing process, the strength of dynamic protective covering also tends to become weak which cannot be restored completely back. Hence the old people usually remain highly susceptibile and when they get exposed to triggering factors they may fall ill. So advanced age can also act as an obstacle.

4) Prolonged other medications: In Homoeopathy the remedy can be slected only after forming the true image of sickness. In order to form this image only the orginal unmodified symptoms that belongs to the patient are taken into consideration. In chronic cases most often the patient turns up to a Homoeopath only as their last resort after taking prolonged continious other school medications. This shall alter the expressions of the orginal symptoms of the true disease. Hence in such cases there can be an obstacle to cure the patient completely. In such cases if the present medication of the patient is not mandatory for the smooth functioning of any vital organs it can be advised to discontinue the present medication and allow the orginal symptoms to

come up after whih a totality can be constructed to form the true picture of the disease.

Difficulties in taking a chronic case

Homoeopathy is well known for uprooting chronic cases. However, taking a chronic case can be very challenging for a homoeopath. Clinically there can be a plenty of difficulties that a Homoeopath may have to encounter while taking a chronic case. Some of these common difficulties are discussed here with a probable solution to overcome such difficulties:

1) Convincing the patient for a detailed case taking: In chronic cases majority of patients turn towards homoeopathy as their last resort. Usually such patients are used to consulting doctors from other school of medicines. The way a homoeopath approaches a case is totally different affair all together. In such cases sometimes it may be difficult to convince the patient for a detailed case taking. The ideal way to overcome this difficulty is to explain and make the patient understand that why a detailed case taking is necessary and what are its benefits.

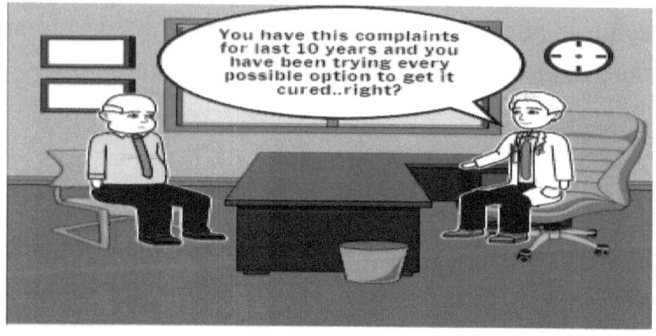
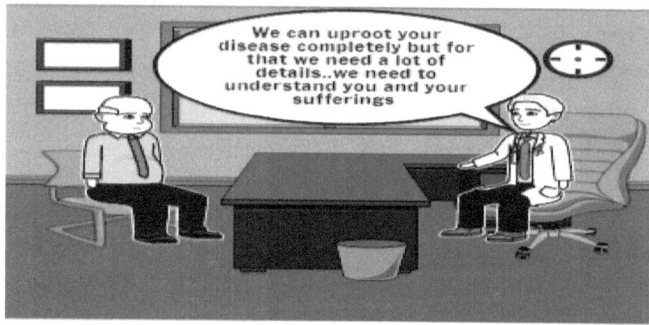
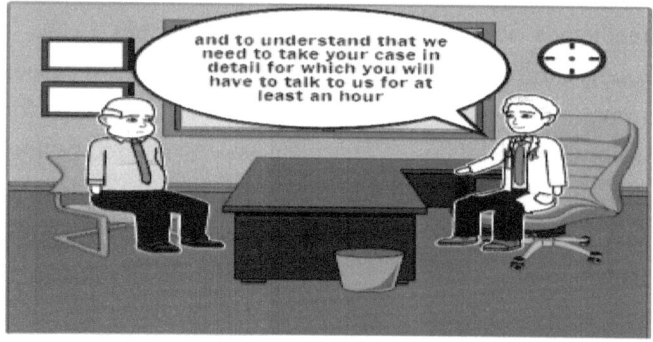

2) Meeting the patient's expectations: Patient's usually do not understand the difference between palliating or giving a temporary relief and removing the

disease completely. Hence even in long standing chronic cases the patient may expect a quick and immediate releif. If they don't feel any better, then there are chances that they may discontinue the medicines and consult other physicians. However, this difficulty also can be overcomed if the patient is made to understand the difference between palliation and complete cure.

3) Tracing the complete image of sickness: Generally chronic diseases are insidious in onset and they tend to progress gradually. In Homoeopathy the remedy can be slected only after forming the true image of sickness which is again constructed on the basis of the orginal unmodified symptoms of the patient. So, in such chronic cases by the time the patient approaches a Homoeopath he may not remember the symptoms that appeared at the time of onset because of his long and continous sufferings. In such cases they only tend to narrate the symptoms which appeared recently. So, it becomes a challenge for the physician to trace the true picture of sickness.

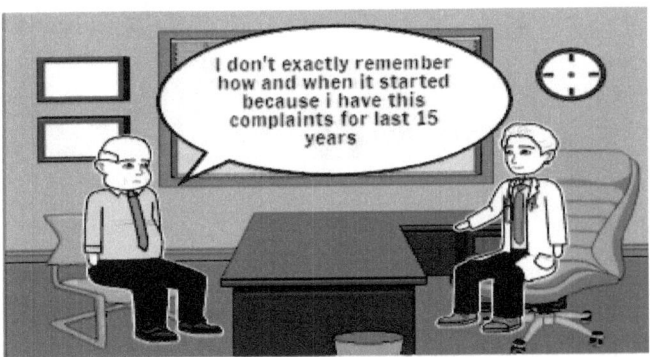

In such cases the patient should be asked to recollect as much as possible the symptoms that existed in the very beginning. Sometimes the information can also be collected from his bystanders who may be able to provide some quality inputs regarding the initial level symptoms.

4) Effect of palliative treatments: Usually in chronic cases the patients turn towards Homeopathy as their last resort especially after taking a prolonged palliative treatment. In such cases the symptoms presented may not belong to the true nature of sickness but may be modfied by such prolonged palliative treatments. As a result, it shall be difficult for a physician to form the true orginal image of sickness.

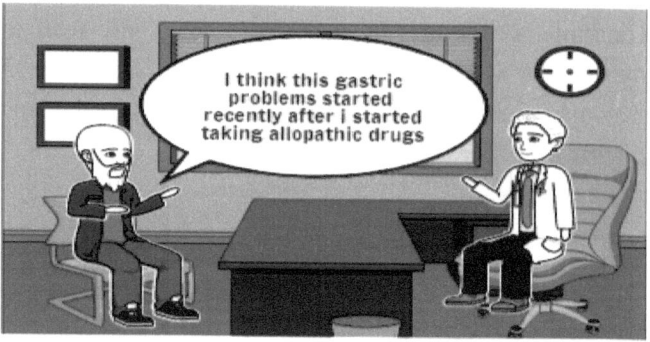

In such cases where the patient is already under other medications it may be advisable to ask the patient to discontinue all such medications provided they are not important for the functioning of any vital organs.

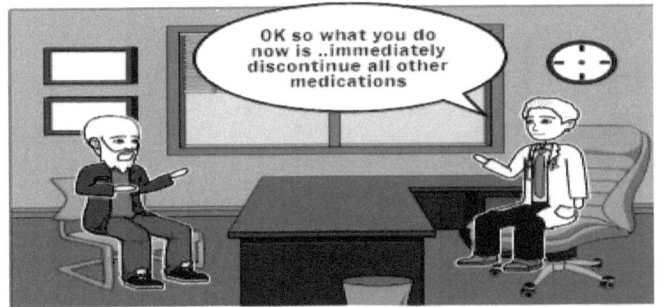

The medicinal symptoms shall seize to exist once such medications are discontinued. The orginal disease symptoms shall then become prominent which can be then grouped together to form the orginal image of sickness.

5) Accessory symptoms not revealed: In many chronic cases because of long standing sufferings patient tends to consider some symptoms as a part of their normal routine life. Such symptoms are called as Accessory symptoms. Usually in clinical practice it is very difficult to trace such symptoms because patients do not reveal those as they consider them to be a part of their normal routine life.

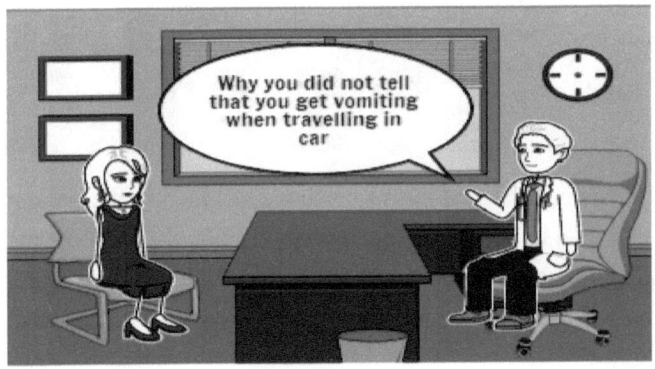

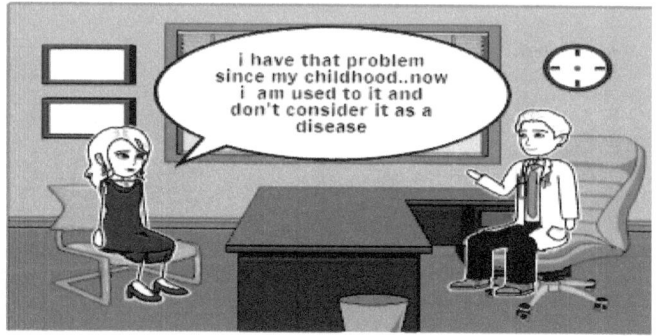

A through and detailed interrogation shall only help to trace out these accessory symptoms. Usally they have a very important role in forming the image of sickness.

6) Patient's coming with diagnostic names of disease: Many patients may consult a homeopath at a stage when the clinical diagnosis has already been made. They tend to come up with such diagnostic names and seek medicines based on their disease name.

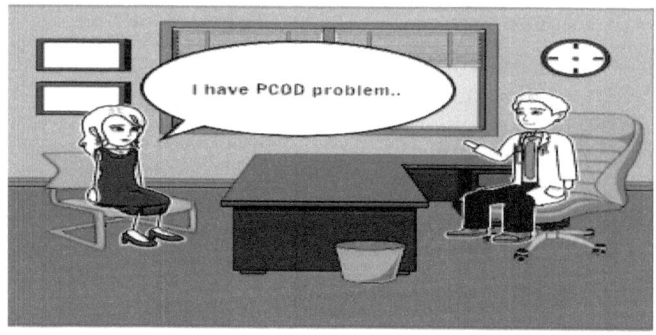

In such cases it has to be first explained to the patient that in Homeopathy the remedy is not decided by the diagnostic name of the disease, but we treat the patient as a whole. The impotance of detailed case taking also has to be explained so that the patient shall then narrate all the informations about him and his complaints.

7) Cases with advanced pathology: It has to be kept in mind that as pathology advances the patients signs and symptoms tends to descrease. So, in cases with advanced pathological changes there may be a scarcity of quality signs and symptoms of the patient. This shall then make it difficult to trace the complete picture of sickness. It is very challenging to overcome this difficulty. However, a detailed interrogation shall help to recover the orginal symptoms that belong to the patient.

8) Hiding symptoms: Some patients tend to hide some information or symptoms that are very personal either because of hesitation or lack of trust upon the physician. These symptoms may either be related to sexual sphere or mental plane and usually are very important for a physician to know.

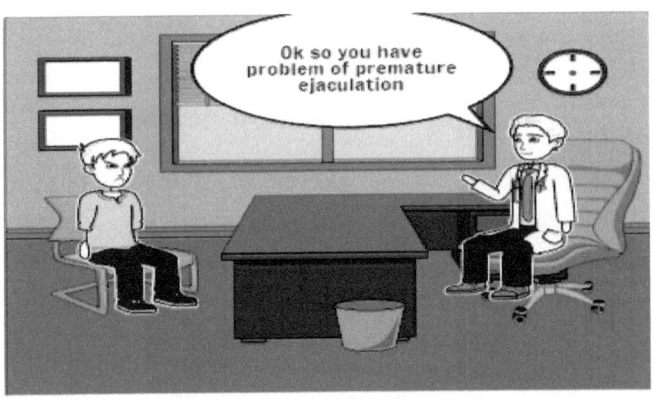

While handling such patients a physician shall first have to ensure that he develops a rapport with the patient. The trust factor has to be build for a smooth flow of information.

9) Alternating symptoms are not revealed: Some group of symptoms tend to alternate with each other. Patients usually do not disclose such alternating symptoms because at the time of consultataion they may probably not remember those as they remain absent at that point of consultataion. Again, a detailed interrogation only shall help to reveal such alternating symptoms.

10) Communication problem: In handling chronic cases of children and old aged people there can be some difficulties in tracing the complete picture of sickness as they may not be able to actively communicate with the physician. In such cases physical examination, keen observation and information collected from the close by-standers of the patient shall help to complete the case.

Homoeopathy as medicine of future:

Homoeopathy has existed for over 200 years but still its true potential in handling acute cases, chronic cases as well as in effective prevention has remained unexplored. Homoeopathy has got several advanatages over the conventional system of medicine.

In acute cases Homoeopathy is the only system which can abort the progress of an acute disease. This means that our remedies have the potential to cure the patient even before the physical symptoms appear. Just consider the below scenario

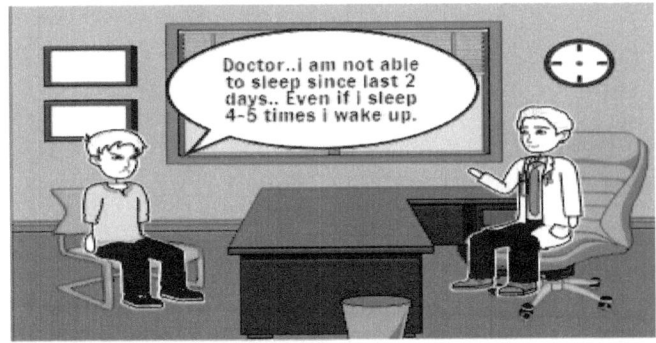

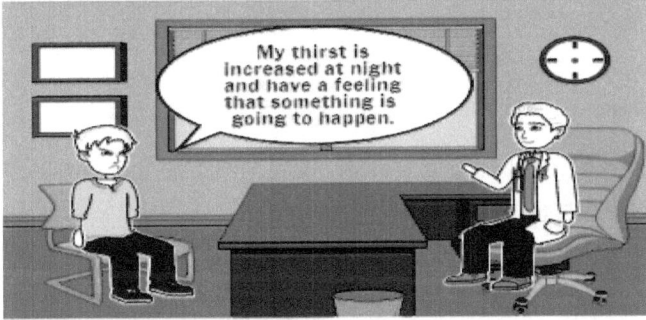

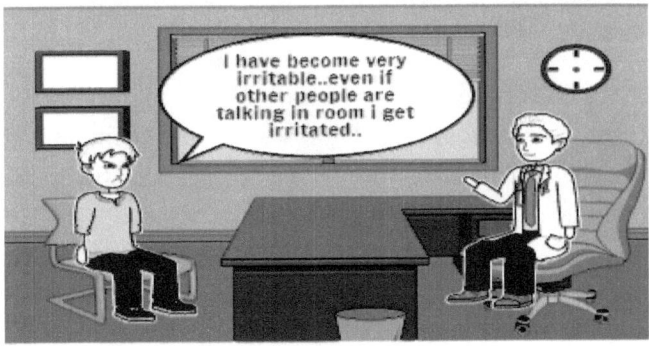

With the above complaints if a patient approaches any other doctor probably, he will be able to do nothing other than to wait for some physical complaints to appear. But a Homoeopath can ensure that the patient is cured even before the physical symptoms appear in such cases.

However, it also has to keep in mind that usually people do not approach a doctor until they develop some physical complaints. This is because of their lack of awareness and if somehow people are made aware as to what is the true potential of Homoeopathy, what to expect from a homoeopath and when to approach him the hidden potential of our remedies can be explored which shall in turn help our system to gain an upper hand as far as handling acute cases are concerned.

Even in those acute cases where the physical symptoms has already appeared a well selected homoeopathic remedy based on the totality and symptoms of the patient shall help to abort the progress of such acute diseases thereby ensuring that the patient is restored back to health in double quick time.

Homoeopathy is well known for handling chronic cases. Even in long standing cases the perfect similimum can completely uproot the disease. This is something that the other school of medicine fails to achieve. We consider the patient as a whole and this wholistic approach not just ensures that the disease is removed but also helps to improve the immune power of the individual.

In cases of epidemics too a well selected homeopathic remedy (genus epidemicus) shall work effectively not only in managing cases of such epidemics but also plays a vital role in active prevention.

How to approach Fever cases

Fever also known as pyrexia or febrile response is a condition where the body's temperature is elevated above its normal range due to an increase in body's temperature set point.

Temperature set point:

The temperature set point is the level at which the body attempts to maintain its temperature. The normal body temperature is aroud 98.5 F. This temperature set point is regulated by the hypothalamus and when this set point is raised the body temperature rises above normal resulting in a condition which is termed as "Pyrexia" or Fever.

It is a routine practice for physicians to advice their patients to take boiled water for drinking. This is because when the water is boiled all the germs, bacterias and other pathogens that may be present in the water gets killed as they fail to survive when the water is boiled thereby making the water sterile for drinking.

Now let's assume a condition wherein the same germs, bacterias or pathogens gains entry into the body (by any means). These pathogens threatens to cause harm and destruction hence needs to be either expelled or killed from the body.

If by rasing the temperature of water (i.e., boiling) the germs, bacterias and other pathogens gets killed then the same logic should apply for our body as well. So, when these pathogens have gained an entry into the body if by any means the body temperature can be raised that shall then make the survival of these pathogens difficult then they shall automatically get killed or expelled. This is what exactly our body does by raising its temperature above the normal limit.

This clearly means that fever is a result of body's defense mechanism. Its an attempt made to kill or expel any source that can pose a threat to cause damage or destruction. So, when a person is having fever it simply means that his body is responding to kill or expel any factors than tend to cause any damage or destruction.

What does anti- pyrectics do

The anti pyretic drugs basically interfere with the body natural defense mechanism and acts to forcibly bring back the temperature set point to normal level for a certain period of time. When the action of such an anti – pyretic drug is exhausted the temperature set point is elevated again and the fever returns. Another dose of such an anti–pyretic drug works in the same fasion to bring down the temperature immediately for a momentarily period of time.

On one hand we have just discussed that the raise in body's temperature is to kill or expel the invaded pathogens so when the temperature is brought down forcibly by interfering with body's normal defense mechanism it in turn faclitates or promotes the growth and multiplication of such invaded pathogens. Hence, we often observe that along with anti-pyretic drugs antibiotics are also prescribed to control or kill the invaded pathogens.

Now the most important question to raise is "does homeopathic remedies act against our body's own self defense mechanism?" if "No" is the answer then what sense it makes by listing fever remedies in Homeopathy? Can homeopathy treat fever or does fever needs to be treated?

Fever is something that needs to be managed and not treated. So, it has to be kept in mind that anti pyretiuc drugs and homeopathic drugs have contrasting actions in cases of fever.

Role of Homeopathic remedies in fever:

Homoeopathic remedies when selected on the basis of totality works in tandem to boost the normal defense mechanism of the body. It has to be kept in mind that unlike the anti pyretics homoeopathic remedies do not work to bring down the temperature alone but it assists the normal defense mechanism to expel, kill or neutrilize the factors that pose a threat to cause damage or destruction thereby resulting in fever. In a well selected remedy shall ensure that the very purpose for which the body has raised its temperature is achieved within one fourth time thereby ensuring that the temperature returns back to normal in much shorter period and the patient recovers in one fourth time. For example, usually in cases of simple viral fevers it shall take around one week for the patient to recover completely. However, under the inflence of a well selected remedy the patient returns back back to health in a day or two.

Basis for selection of Homoeopathic remedy in fever

Just like in other cases in fevers too the remedy has to be selected based on the totality. This totality is constructed on the basis of quality symptoms of the patient and not of the disease. No two cases of fever can be exactly alike. The individual reactions may vary, the alterations may vary too and similarily the presenting individualistic symptoms shall also vary. So, based on this individualistic symptoms or characteristic modalities the remedy has to be selected.

Do we have painkillers in Homoeopathy?

Let's first try to understand as to how and why do we feel pain. In response to a trauma or injury, a person feels pain once the affected cells have reacted to it.

Let's see how it works

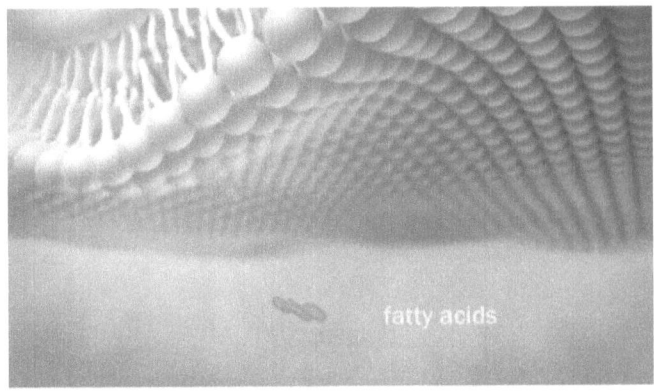

In case of Injury or trauma the cell membrane of the affected cells immediately release fatty acids. These fatty acids enter an enzyme called cyclo-oxygenase present on the cell membrane.

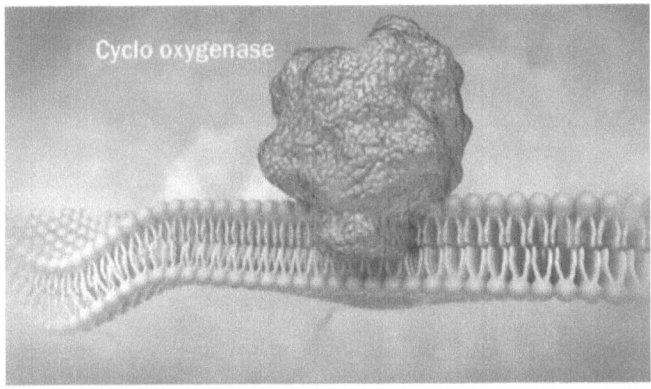

They are then converrted into pain messenger substances. These pain messenger substances then go and fit into the pain receptors present on the nerve endings thereby stimulating it.

This stimulation generates an electrical signal which is sent to the brain. Brain receives this information and evaluates it and then the person feels pain. This entire process occurs within just few seconds.

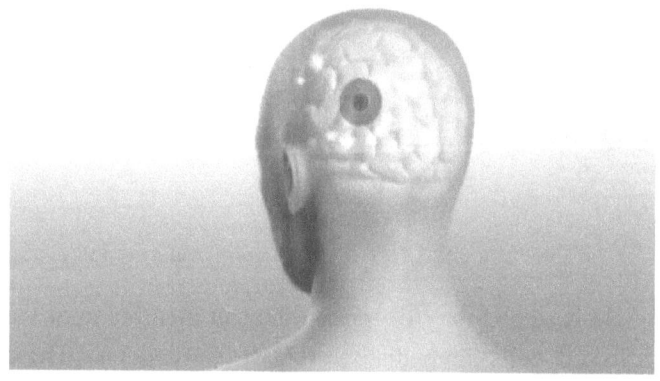

Now if we wish to kill this pain there are 3 ways:

1) By preventing the damaded or injured cells from releasing fatty acids: This cannot be done by any means as long as the cell is living.

2) By blocking the fatty acids from entering the cyclo-oxygenase enzyme thereby preventing these fatty acids from getting converted into pain messenger cells. This is exactly how these allopathic pain killers works. Here it has to be kept in mind that by doing so there is an interference into the functioning of body's self defense mechanism.

3) By blocking the electrical transmission from nerve endings reaching the brain. Again, by this means too we are directly interfering with the normal body's self defense mechanism.

Now the most improtant question is can Homoeopathic remedies act against the body's self defense mechanism?

If "No" then does it make sense by listing remedies as pain killers in Homeopathy?

Pain is a part of body's self defense mechanism indicating that something is not right in that concerned part or around it from where this pain stimulus is generated. It also helps to keep that affected part under attention and rest which is equally essential for recovery and restoration.

If a person is feeling the pain stimulus there has to be a cause and if we could remove this cause the outcome which is in the form of pain shall automatically disappaear.

Homoeopathic remedy aims at giving that additional push to the vital force to assist it in removing the cause. For doing so again the remedy has to be slected on the basis of individual totality.

Role of Homoeopathic remedies in Mechanical trauma

Mechanical trauma is an injury to any portion of the body from a blow, crush, cut, or penetrating wound. From the definition it is very clear that this is something that is realted and limited only to the materialistic plane.

If we refer the 10th aphorism (Organon 6th edition) it states *"The material organism, without the vital force, is capable of no sensation, no function, no self-preservation, it derives all sensation and performs all the functions of life solely by means of the immaterial being (the vital principle) which animates the material organism in health and in disease."*

It is very clear from the above aphorism that the vital force when in order is responsible for protection and self preservation. Self preservation also includes repair of damaged or injured parts. So, when the vitality is in order it shall ensure that the trauma or mechanical injuries limited only to the materiastic plane shall be automatically reparied by the vital force. Hence no medical aid is necessary in cases of mechanical injuries as they tend to heal off by its own. To quote from the literature:

"If man is injured from the external, e.g., if he has his finger torn, it will soon be repaired; the order which is in the economy from centre to circumference will repair every wrong that is on the surface caused by external violence." (J T Kent)

However, in serious and grave injuries or mechanical displacements or disoreintations and fractures the help of a surgeon is needed to fix the issue. In such cases the vitality is disturbed but not deranged. Hence homoepathic remedies has a limited role to play. Here, is the reference:

"He who has a lacerated wound, or a broken bone, or deformities, has need of a surgeon. If his tooth must come out he must have a surgeon dentist.

What would be thought of a man who, on being sent for a surgeon to set an injured man's bones should go for a carpenter to mend the roof of the man's house?

If the man's house alone needs mending then he needs a carpenter and not a surgeon. The physician must discriminate between the man and his house, and between the repair of man and repair of his house.

It is folly to give medicine for a lacerated wound, to attempt to close up a deep wound with a dose of remedy.

Injuries from knives, hooks, etc., affect the house the man lives in and must be attended to by the surgeon." (J T Kent)

Role of placebos in Homoeopathy

Placebo is also known as the second-best remedy in Homoeopathy. This in itself highlights the importance of them in Homeopathic practice. What do these placebos contain? Why it is known as the second-best remedy?

Its usually said and believed that palcebos only have a psychological effect. Can this psychological effect alone have an impact upon the health of a person?

The psychological effect has a dynamic influence upon a person and can be of two types:

1) Negtive

2) Positive

Here are some examples of negative psychological effects:

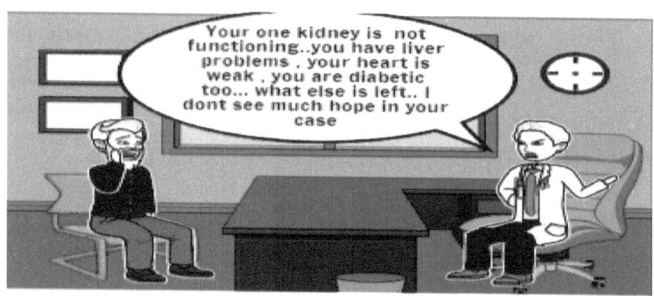

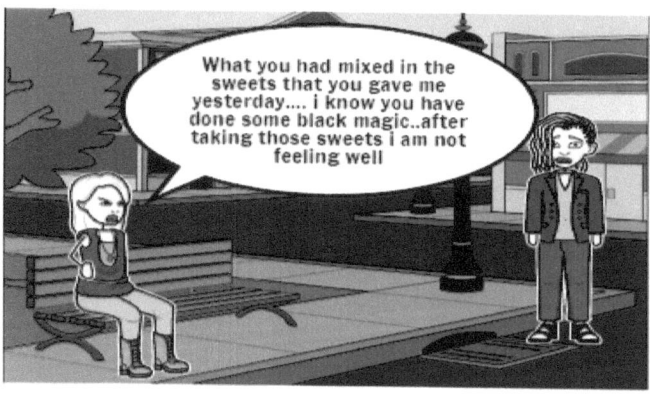

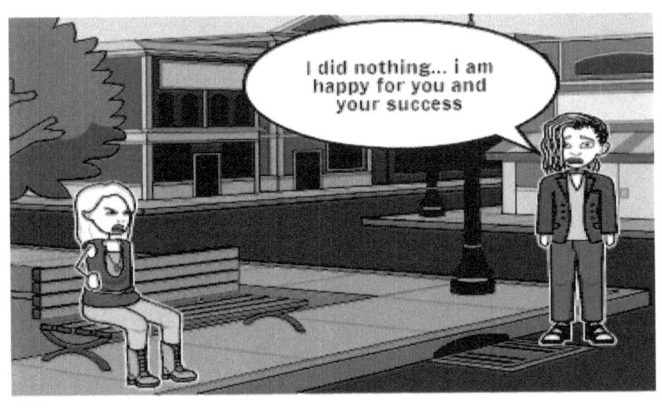
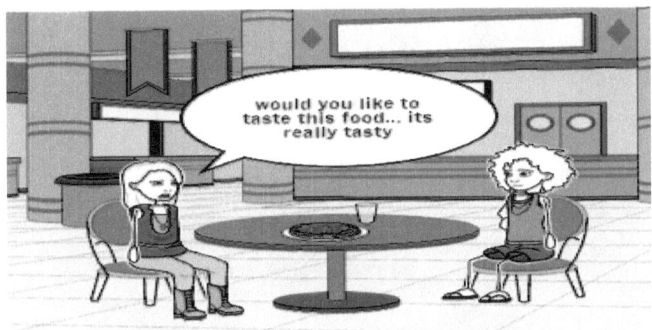
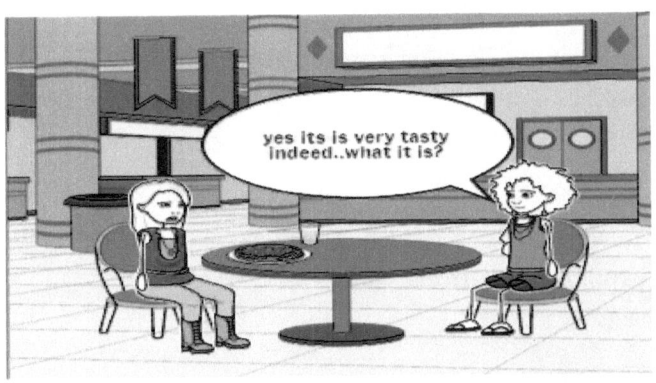

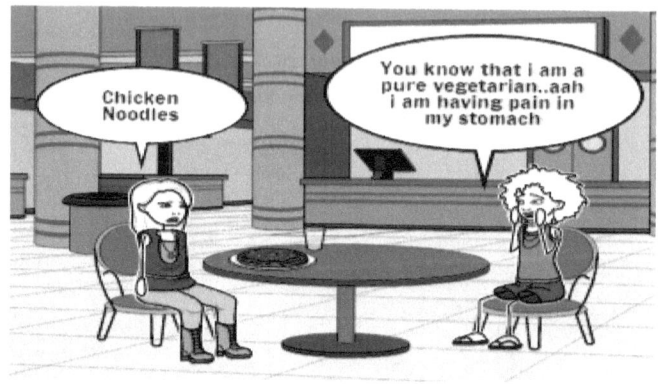

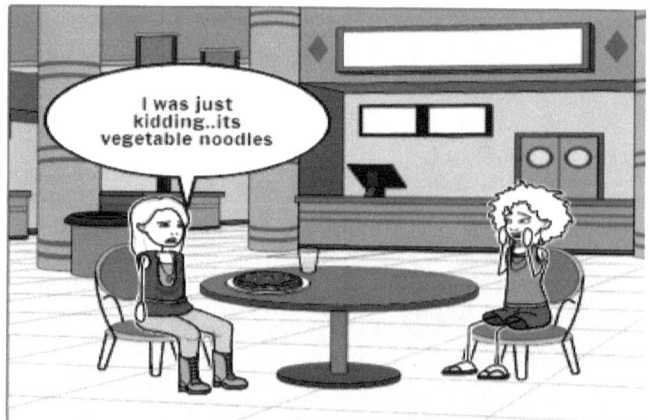

As it can be seen from the above examples negative psychological effect has a negative impact upon the body at a dynamic level and can contribute to make a person feel sick.

Now let's consider some examples of Positive psychological effects:

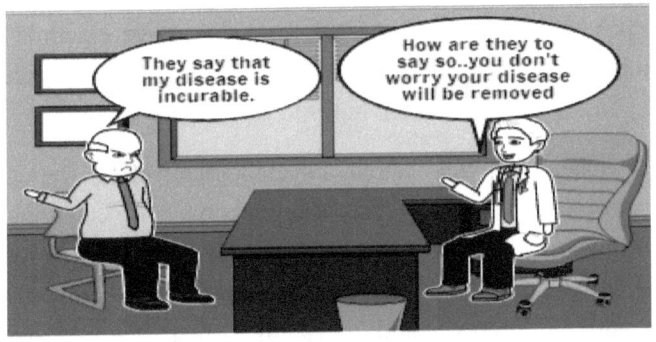
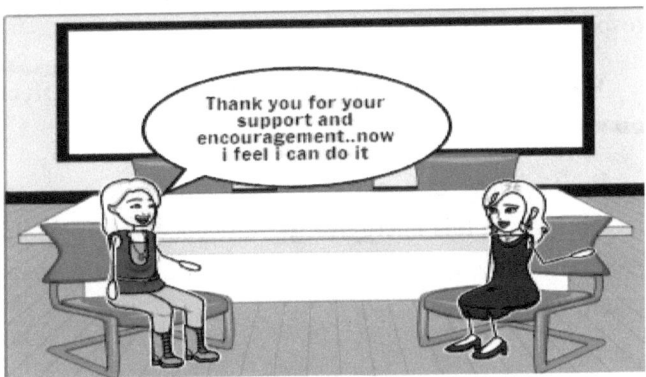
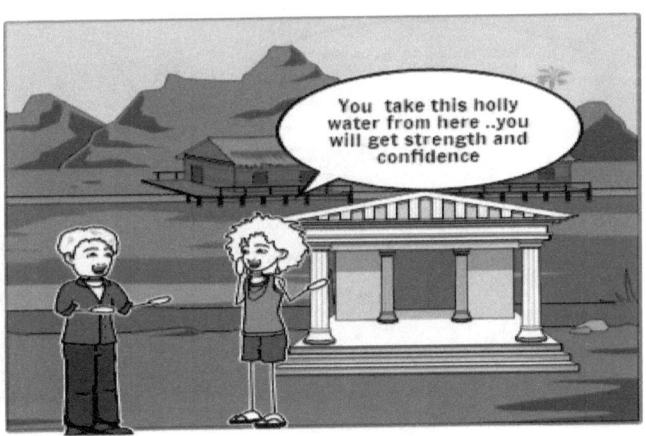

As it can be clearly seen from the above examples that positive psychological effects have a positive impact upon the body and often helps to cure a person.

When we talk about psychological effect be it positive or negative it is the outcome of something influencing the body at a dynamic level to bring about such effects. Thius something is what we called dynamic positive energy and dynamic negative energy respectively.

Why does these energies do not have same effect on all?

Be it positive or negative dynamic influence a person has to receive this energy to get influenced by it. Mind plays a deciding role in this matter. Below are some examples:

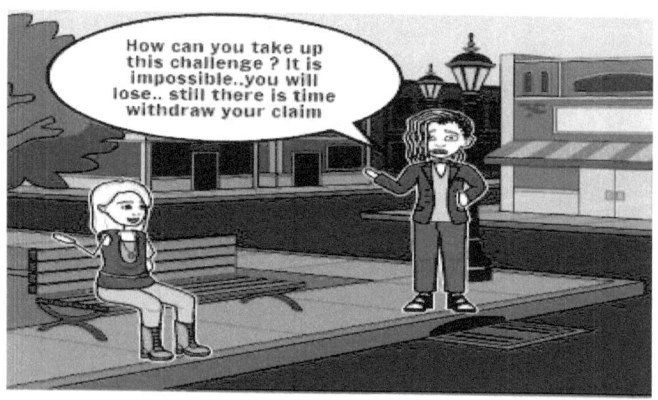

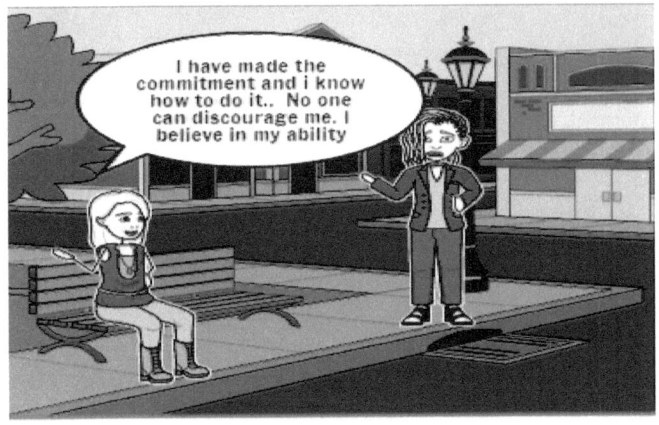

As you can see from the above example that the negative energy in the form of discouragement is not affecting at all the other person because her will power is strong enough not to accept or receive such negative vibes. On the other hand, have a look at the example given below:

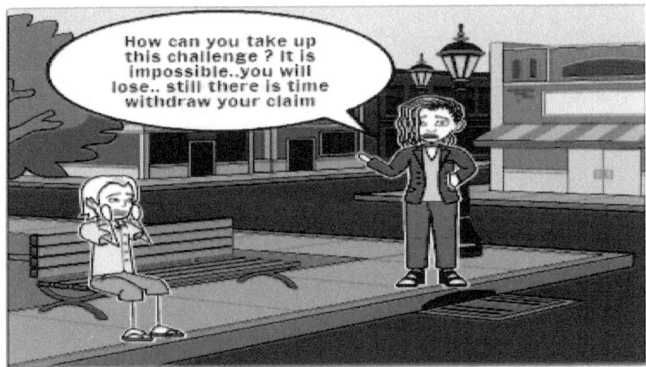

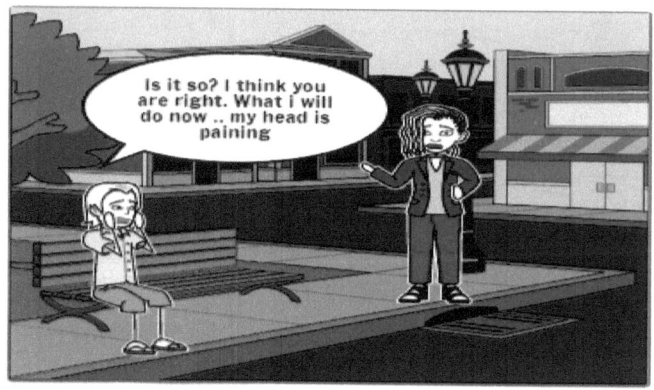

As you can see from the above example as to how the negative energy can influence the person at a dynamic level when she is in receiving mode and can cause a derangement in health.

If negative vibes or energies acting at a dynamic level can make a person sick, then positive vibes or energies acting at the same level shall contribute towards curing a person.

Can this positive phychological effect alone can cure a person: To understand this let's consider an example

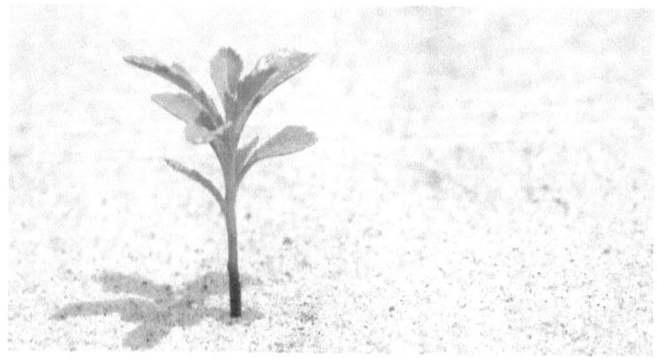

The above images show a very small tiny plant. It shall be very easy to uproot this plant using just one one finger as this task shall require only a minimum energy. Now consider the image given below:

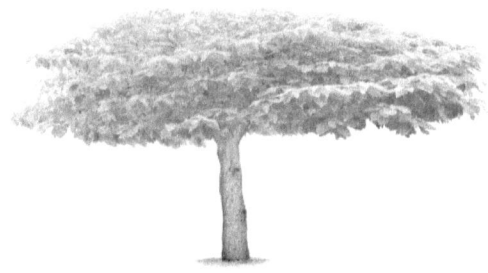

If the above tree has to be uprooted it canot be done using a finger or a hand as in this case it is much deep rooted and strong and hence requires more energy to uproot it.

Same is the case with diseases too. Some minor alterations in health caused by any negative dynamic influence can sometimes be eliminated and vitality can be restored back to health without the aid of any medicines but only with a little positive dynamic energy or influence. Here is a clinical example:

Step by step approach to practice classical homoeopathy

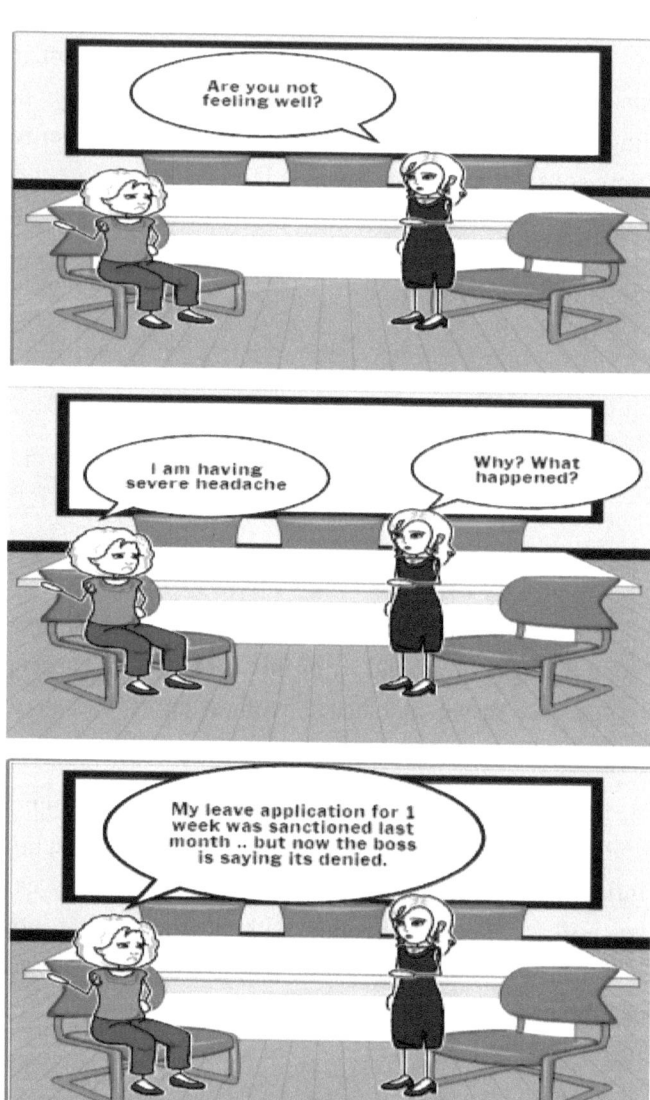

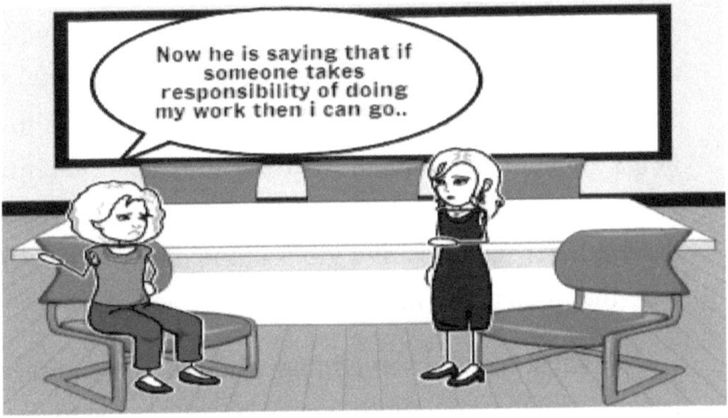

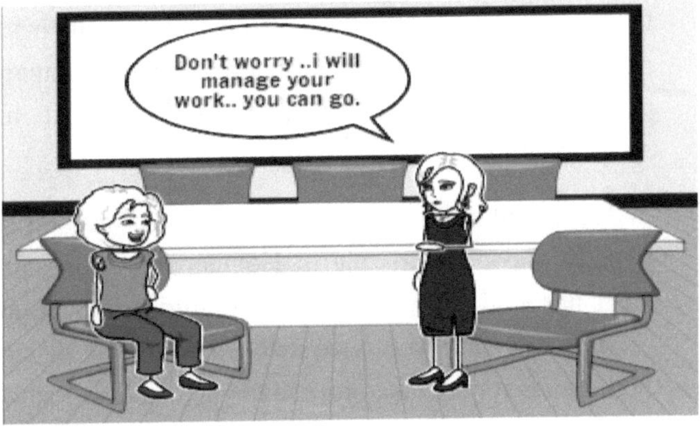

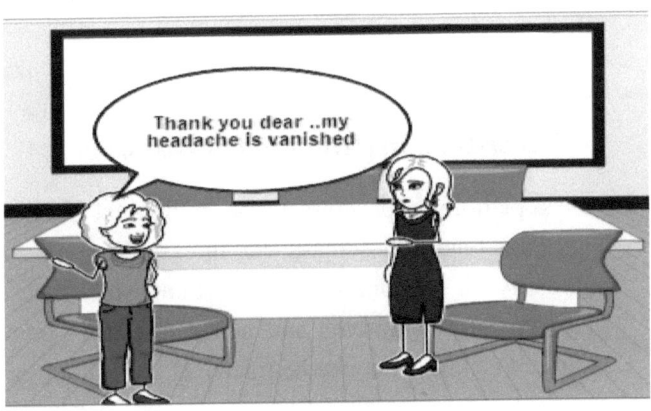

In such trivial deviations from health even without any medical aid the positive energy recived from any source can help to restore the vitality back to health and helps to cure the patient without the help of remedy. However, in cases where the vitality is deranged to a drastic level such positive vibes alone may not be able to cure the patient and remedy would be needed.

We must have observed that when the patient has the trust on doctor sometimes even placebos helps to cure as these palcebos contain the positive energy which has a positive phychological effect upon the patient imparting positive energy which acts at dynamic level to bring about the cure.

Hence placebos also known as the second best remedy plays a vital role in Homeopathy. Also, as Dr Kent has said *"Never be in a hurry to prescribe for a chronic case until you have understood the whole case"*. Sometimes it may take more than one consultation to get this whole picture. Till the mean time the patient can be kept on placebos to gain the positive phychological effect.

Prescribing in pathological cases:

As pathology progresses the individual signs and symptoms tend to descrease. So, in cases with advanced pathology it becomes very difficult to trace the individualistic symptoms and hence true and complete nature of sickness may be be traced. If the pathology has extended to cause an irreversible damage, then in such cases palliation is the only option left. The remedy can then be selected based on the prominent particular symptoms.

However, it has to be kept in mind that pathology relates to the disease and not to the person. Among such pathological changes if we can observe something that is strange and peculiar then those set of symptoms require special attention.

At the same time if same kind of pathological changes are observed at more than one part then such changes becomes a characteristic feature belonging to that particular individual. Such group of symptoms is called pathological generals. They usually have high value in slecting a remedy.

In cases where along with pathology prominent generals are traceable then more importance should be given to the generals.

As Dr Kent has said *"The man who waits for pathology to guide him to a remedy for a constitutional sickness is most unwise.*

We sometimes see the remedy shining through the pathology, but generally only the smallest hints are visible. These hints may strengthen the indications, but it is better to strengthen the indications with the early symptoms.".

Polypharmacy or prescribing multiple remedies:

This is the most common way of prescribing that majority of us follow. Although such practices have been severely condemned in our literature still we opt for this kind of prescriptions under the sweet name of Modernization and experience. How fair it is to prescribe more than one remedy at a time? Does this kind of prescription makes any sense?

We all know that Homeopathy is based on the principle of "Similia similibus curanter" where we believe that the indicated remedy shall produce similar by stronger symptoms that already exist in the patient thereby removing the orginal symptom.

Now when we prescribe two or more remedies how shall we acertain that which remedy shall act to produce the existing symptoms in the patient? If more than one indicated remedy has the potential to produce the orginal symptom that exists in the patient, then in such a situation which remedy shall produce it and who will decide that?

For example, if a patient having sour ercutations along with other complaints is prescribed both Nux vomica and carbo veg then which remedy shall produce this sour ercutations to remove the orginal symptom as both these remedies has the potential to produce this symptom and on what basis that will be decided?

If it is argued that any one shall produce, then do we mean to say that the remedies have that self intelligence to decide for themselves as to which symptoms to produce? If so, then why is it needed to take the case in detail and form the totality? We can easily prescribe a set of remedies they shall then decide among themselves.

If we say that both remedies shall act, then it should be taken for granted that if two remedies can act together even 200 remedies can do so as well. Does that make sense?

So, people may even say that our remedies act upon the vital force so the vital force shall decide as to which remedy shall act. Now if this is considered to be true then we can think of making a master remedy by combining all the proven remedies available. The vital force shall then decide for itself as to which remedy it needs.

In short, all such arguments make no sense and the entire basic foundation of Homeopathy and its principles severily condemn and discard the use of multiple remedies.

One-line prescribers:

There are some people who base their prescription on one or two symptoms. Such one-line prescriptions cannot be justified as in Homeopathy the remedy is selected based on the totality and not on any one or two individual symptoms. It has to be kept in mind that presence of one symptom does not rule in favor of a remedy nor absence of one rule out a remedy. It's the totality that decides the final selction. All those who claim to have got results with such one-line prescriptions are doing nothing but trying their luck upon their patients. Such results are nothing more than a "Lucky Hit".

"Many cases are presented with no generals and no mental symptoms - absolutely no characterizing symptoms - only the symptoms common to sickness. When a successful prescription is made on such symptoms, it is scarcely more than a "lucky hit" (J T Kent)"

Keynote prescription:

Keynote symptoms are those peculiar symptoms in a case that shall help to find out a small group of remedies.

Such keynotes symptoms often have a high value in forming the totality. They shall in many cases give a clear indication towards a remedy. However, it has to be kept in mind that ideally these keynote symptoms alone should not form the base of prescription. They when go together with the other generals of the case shall help to confirm the selection.

"There are strange and rare symptoms, even in parts of the body, which the experienced physician learns are

so guiding that they must be ranked in the higher and first classes. These include some keynotes which may guide safely to a remedy or to the shaping of results, provided that the Mental and the physical generals do not stand contrary, as to their modalities, and therefore oppose the keynote symptoms." J T kent

From the above phrase it's very clear that keynote symptoms shall definitely help to shortlist a group of remedies provided the mental and physical generals do not oppose such keynote symptoms by indicating towards another remedy.

Again, the keynote symptoms listed under a drug need not necessiarily have the same importance in the patient. Say for example the keynote symptoms of Bryonia are

1) Aggravation from least motion
2) Dryness of mucus membrane
3) Excessive thirst

Now if a patient is in a severily dehydrated state then all the above listed keynotes becomes normal for such a patient. Hence, they lose their value. For such cases if bryonia is indicated may end up in failure.

"A keynote prescriber is but a memory prescriber; he has memorised only and has not made it a part of his understanding. Such prescribers are almost useless, and it is among them that we find "falling from grace" (J T kent)

Listing remedies for clinical conditions:

We often see people listing remedies for various clinical conditions like best remedies for asthma, arthritis, migraine etc. How fair it is to make such listings? Do such listings make sense?

"Every few days I run across a homoeopathic physican who asks: "What remedy are you using in such and such case?"

Such a thing has no place in my mind, and I look upon one who speaks in that way as a man untrained in homoeopathics.

I truly have lost my patient over such things, for the old gray-heads, who have practiced for years and pretended to practice Homeopathy, do not hestitate to say that "the best remedy for epilepsy" is so and so. What a nonsense!" (Lecture no. 9; Lectures on homoeopathic philosophy-J T Kent)

It becomes very clear from the above phrase that no such listings made in homeopathy make sense. In homeopathy we treat the disease and not the disease ultimates. Asthma, arthritis, migraine etc are not diseases but they are the disease ultimates i.e., the endings. Literature further says *"Every remedy has in itself a certain state of peculiarities that identifies it as an individual remedy, and the patient has also a certain state of peculiarities that identifies him as an individual patient, and so the remedy is fitted to the patient.*

No remedy must be given because it is in the list, for the list has only been made as a means of facilitating the study of that epidemic" (Lecture no. 3; Lectures on homoeopathic philosophy-J T Kent)

Now, its very clear from the above phrase that for a remedy to fit in as the similimum for a given case the peculiarities of the remedy must match with the peculiarities of the patient. These individual peculiarities vary from person to person. So, how can a remedy which may seem to have worked for a given condition in a patient shall be expected to produce the same result in every individual suffering from the same clinical condition?

The individual peculiarities differ from person to person and hence the remedy shall also change based on these peculiarities.

Managing surgical cases:

Homoeopathy has a great potential in managing successfully even some of the cases that requires surgery. It can help to cure the patient in a much shorter span of time thereby avoiding the need for a surgery. Cases like uterine fibroids, calculi, tumors etc can be managed with the help of a perfectly selected similimum.

It has to be kept in mind that even in such surgical cases the remedy has to be selected based on the totality of sysptoms. Also, at the same time it has to be kept in mind that all cases that may need a surgery cannot be handled with Homeopathy. In cases like displacements, dislocations and severe mechanical trauma or injury indeed needs to be handled by a surgeon.

In cases which can be fatal if not immediately handled by surgical means also falls under the limitations of Homeopathy.

Defective books and defective use of books:

In his lesser writings Dr J.T. Kent has said that *"Homoeopathy is slow to win its way because of the defective use of books, as well as because of defective books, thus producing results that are not striking but merely ordinary."*

Homoeopathy has the potential to yield extraordinary results. Such results can be obtained only when we learn to stick to the basic laws, theories and principles. Unfortunately, this is the major defect with many of us.

When we talk about this defectiveness it can be a result of

a) Using defective books

b) Defective use of books

Using defective books in the sense those books which serve baseless short cuts, tips, remedy suggestions based on allopathic mode of prescribing, easy listing of remedies etc. Such books are plenty in market today which hinder the growth of our system. Just a litle logical thinking is required to decide the fate of such books. For a moment let's imagine that such books are efficient and useful in giving results clinically in majority of cases. If that was the case, then by now we should have been able to put an end to the critics and allegations that we are facing.

The fact is such books can give one results that looks ordinary and are not consistent too. They only serve to make your task easy at the cost of doing great harm to your patients and to our entire system.

Defective use of books in the sense, utilizing the books not in order with the guidelines based on which a book is compiled. Let's take the example of using Kent's repertory. Majority of us just randomly take out a few observed symptoms in the patient and feed it into the repertory and expect the repertory to do the rest and come up with the similimum. This is defective use of book. Kent's repertory has its own philosophical background and the book has to be used accordingly i.e., by constructing a perfect totality that fits in with its philosophy.

Value of experience:

Experience has a great value in Homeopathy. As Dr Kent has said "Prescribing the homoeopathic remedy is such a process of growth and progress that it may be said that "the best of the wine is saved for the last of the feast." Along with this progress a physician shall become rich in his experience and a master in performing his task to its perfection.

With this ever growing experience a physician shall attain perfection in applying the laws clinically for serving the people and humanity. He gains a firm belief in the laws and principles of Homeopathy as he shall witness them clinically getting confirmed with each confrontation with the patient.

"It is well to hope-for all to hope that, with experience, each may attain the high degree of perfection in healing that Hahnemann attained." (Chapter 3; Lesser writings - J T kent)

It is a fact that prescribing becomes easier with experience. However, this experience can be of any good only when it shall confirm the law. Today we see that a lot of so-called experienced physicians resort to the years of experience they own as an excuse to deviate from the law and make their own rules in order to make their prescription easy. Such experiences are of no use if it goes against the law.

A path has been laid by our masters and our experience if going in right direction can only confirm the path to be true and trustworthy.

"They who practice on a part of Hahnemann's teachings and fill the great void with "results of experience," do so with methods that the master unequivocally condemned; and while it may not be thought kindly of the statement is true; they are not the homoeopathists who have followed in the footsteps of the master." (Chapter 30; Lesser writings-J T Kent)

Experience has a place in science, but only a confirmatory place. It can only confirm that which has been discovered through principle or law guiding in the proper direction.

Experience leads to no discoveries, but when man is fully indoctrinated in principle that which he observes by experience may confirm the things that are consistent with law.

One who has no doctrines, no truth, no law, who do not rely upon law for everything, imagines he discovers by experience.

Out of his experience he undertakes to invent, and his inventions runs in every conceivable direction ; hence we may see in this centuary a medical convention of a thousand physicians who entirely upon experience, at which one will arise and relate his experience, and another will arise and tell his experience, and the talkers of that convention continue to debate and no two talkers agree.

When they are finished they compare their experiences and that which they settle upon they call science, no matter how far they may be from the truth.

Next year they come back and they have different ideas and have had different experiences, and they then vote out what they voted in before.

This is the medicine of experience.

They confirm nothing, but make from experience a series of inventions and theories. This is the wrong direction.

The science of medicine must be build on a true foundation. (Lecture 4; Lectures on Homoeopathic philosophy - J T Kent)

Instead of taking the critics in a wrong way we all should sit and think "What are we doing to our patients and to our system by following the same methodologies which has already been condemned in our literature under the sweet name of experience and modernization? What value does such an experience has when it doesn't confirm the law.

Consistency is the key:

Consistency in giving results is the key to sort out all the controversies and put an end to the critics and allegations that Homoeopathy has been facing till date. This consistency can be achieved only when we all learn to accept our master as the final authority and stick to the instructions and guidelines given in the organon and philosophy.

Today we lack this consistency because we have got diverted from the path and either because of our own ignorance and self ego or for our own ease we have buried the laws theories and principles on the basis of which our system was once build.

It's high time for us to excavate those buried theories laws and principles to take our system to a level where Homeopathy shall be the number one choice among the common people when it comes to serving their healthcare needs.

Reference

- Organon of medicine (6th edition) by Dr. Samule Hahnemann
- Lectures on homoeopathic philosophy by J.T. Kent,
- Lesser writings by J.T. Kent

Epilogue

Step by step approach to practice classical Homeopathy is just a guide that can be of help if one wish to follow the right path. The path that gives a consistency in our clinical practicethe path that builds our confidence with ech and every case and the path that shall bring success and glory not just to individual Homoeopaths but to our entire system as well.

As Dr Kent has said "The inexperienced must be assisted and instructed in order to practice Homoeopathy without resort to traditional medicine. But assistance can be of use only when desired and appreciated."

This book compilation is for those who desires that assiastance and appreciates it. It shall throw only a light on to the correct path and each and every one who wishes to follow the right path has to do so putting in their best efforts. They have to travel this journey at their own pace. This book shall only guide and ensure that the path is maintained.

For any feedbacks or queries related to the contents mentioned in this book kindly drop an email to uers15@gmail.com

www.ingramcontent.com/pod-product-compliance
Lightning Source LLC
Chambersburg PA
CBHW020730180526
45163CB00001B/185